REFLECTING

CONTINUING CIRCULAR EMAILS FROM A COUNTRY VICAR DURING THE PANDEMIC

Kingsley Taylor

Grosvenor House
Publishing Limited

This book is published by
Grosvenor House Publishing Ltd
Link House
140 The Broadway, Tolworth, Surrey, KT6 7HT.
www.grosvenorhousepublishing.co.uk

A CIP record for this book
is available from the British Library

ISBN 978-1-83975-627-6

Dedication

To Jo-an who continues to support and encourage me and keep me sane in these strange times.

Contents

Preface

I finished my last book at a hopeful time when restrictions were slowly being lifted and the numbers of deaths were dropping. But it was not over and we were warned of a second wave. So I continued to write these daily emails. The second wave came and this was worse than the first, we had a second and a third lockdown. I continued to try and give hope as people became more frightened and weary. As Easter approached the second wave eased, some restrictions were lifted and more people were being vaccinated we began to hope again. So I end this book at a hopeful time too, having been able to celebrate Easter this year.

As I have always maintained these are not thoughts for the day, people have found them encouraging, amusing and wise but in essence they are only the daily ramblings of a country Vicar during the pandemic. I write on ...

Acknowledgement

This is a pilgrimage that many of us have been on together and I want to thank all who have come with me, we have learned so much together.

Part 1
Slow Easing

Tue 4 Aug

Subject: LMA the sequel

Dear Friends

There are a lot of butterflies about. Creatures that had been stomping about and eating leaves closed themselves up into chrysalises shut off from the world. Now they are butterflies, and it was good to see so many butterflies in the churchyard of St Mary's on Sunday. The joy of butterflies meeting up again and seeing each other again. This was a good statement to the world, people had been remarking about it in the paper shop and quite likely other places as well. I have heard from other butterflies that weren't there physically but were there spiritually anyway.

Where do we go from here? We go forward with God as our guide with joy and hope and a spring in our steps (and wings). Have you seen the size of butterfly wings that are big enough to lift a being our size?

God be with you

Kingsley

Wed 5 Aug

Subject: LMA follow up

Dear Friends

In one of my earlier emails I commented on what was normal. Before Jesus met the disciples they had normal lives, then following him was normal, then after his death and resurrection was another normal, then after the ascension when they went out into the world was another normal again. With us our old normal was brought suddenly to an end with the lockdown, and that was the new normal, our present normal is the slow easing of restrictions and it changes week by week. So I ask again, what is normal?

There is no real normal, life changes all the time and always has done. The life of a child changes from being at home to going to school, changing from one school to another, taking exams, going to work, having a family and watching them grow up, and so on. Life is a process, a journey. For us who have been living through unusual times it has only highlighted this anyway. Life is about new experiences, seeing new things, meeting new people, it is an adventure. Each of us has a story that is personal to us.

We do not yet know what today holds (well the rest of today anyway) and tomorrow is another day. Live each day with expectation and excitement.

Regards

Kingsley

Thu 6 Aug

Subject: LMA supplement

Dear Friends

Does everyone have times when you feel you must go somewhere or telephone someone and you have no idea where that has come from and you find you have done exactly the right thing at the right moment? You can go out of your way for someone and they will hardly notice or expect it as a right while other people you can do something so simple you don't even think about it and their appreciation is so profuse it takes you by surprise. It is a funny world isn't it. Well perhaps not the world but the people in it. Perhaps it is the difference between when we respond to pressures from outside or when we listen to the little voice within.

God only seems to speak in a little voice, so little we don't realise it is him.

Kingsley

Fri 7 Aug

Subject: continuation

Dear Friends

We had to go to Carmarthen again, it was easier this time. After the necessary we went to Costa for a coffee but they were full so we popped across to Tiger we went all round before coming to look for the thing we were after and the girl behind the counter said they didn't have any before we even started to look, she recognised us and knew what we were looking for with all the people who must go in to Tiger and it was five months since we were last there. We went back to Costa just as some people were coming out so we could go in and sit at a table to have our coffee, as I ordered two skinny lattes the girl said one is extra extra hot, again with all the people who go into Costa and with us not having been there for five months she knew that Jo-an liked her coffee really hot. Later in Morrisons Jo-an had her mask on and a woman who had served in a couple of shops in Carmarthen recognised her and had a chat. The personal touch, people remembering you, isn't it so much better than technology!

God knows us all by name, he knows us better than we know ourselves, isn't it great to know that God is not some remote being who is not really interested in us. When he speaks to us it is personal not general.

Hear God speak to you today

Kingsley

Sat 8 Aug

Subject: LMA etcetera

Dear Friends

One thing I never have been able to grasp is hierarchy, why one person should be more important because they have a title. I understand it as an organisational structure but because people have different jobs doesn't make them better, it is who a person is that counts. I understand also that certain positions require a certain training that may take a few years, but it is what individuals do with the training that matters. The disciples had three years training with Jesus, then forty days intensive preparation after his resurrection, and they still had compassion on the crippled and the bereaved, with their training came a responsibility to care for people and to spread the gospel. I often refer back to the Celtic Church where you couldn't always tell which one was the bishop because he (or she) would just as likely be tilling the ground, dropping in on sick people unannounced, as presiding over a group of clergy and laity. The church did have a structure but it was much more free and informal. And this is what we need now, we need everyone, clergy and laity on an equal footing to be the church in the community and this is what I have seen more and more even before the lockdown.

We all have good news and we show this in our lives and our dealings with people, we are the church.

Kingsley

Sun 9 Aug

Subject: LMA Trinity 9

Dear Friends

Matthew 14:22-33. After feeding five thousand Jesus at last has a chance to be alone, you remember he is still grieving for John the Baptist, so he sent his disciples back in the boat. As they are crossing the wind whips up and he is not there to calm the storm. Then they spot calmly walking on the water. Peter (always the rash one) wants to walk on the water too and he actually does for a while until he notices the wind and the waves. As he sinks Jesus saves him and the wind dies down. They realise he is the Son of God, well at that point anyway, but he says nothing.

Some people like the sound of their own voice and will go on for ages, or is it that they think the more words they use the more the other person is enlightened. I am afraid one of my greatest failings is a short attention span, my mind just switches off and I hope I get the point when they get to it. In a lengthy email I just scroll to the bottom. My apologies to anyone who has thought they had my full attention. Jesus said what he needed to say in as few words as possible, and very often in a story never a lecture. Has anyone read Don Black's 'The Sanest Guy in the Room'? I'm with Don.

Kingsley

Mon 10 Aug

Subject: LMA Week 20

Dear Friends

I am still trying to analyse how I felt yesterday having had a service inside St Mary's after so long. There is, as I have often said, a sense of peace there, not only is there an angel but it is the centuries of prayer (unbroken until recently) that have taken place there. I know you can pray anywhere but there you can almost feel the combined prayer of all the people who have ever prayed there. I also felt a sense of arriving, of returning almost fulfilment. Worship is a corporate thing, when we make the effort to come together and share worship it has that extra dimension. The only thing that was sadly lacking was singing. Sitting here in front of my computer tapping away does not replace seeing your faces and gauging your responses, though I am grateful for all the responses you have given me by return of email. Not being able to see people is also one of the reasons I could not do a service at home and send it out over the internet, that and my stone age understanding of technology.

For God so loved the world that he gave his one and only Son. (Jn 3:16a). This is what marks Christianity as different from every other religion, we do not have a remote God but a God with us, and he asks us to follow his example. I am happiest when I can be with people and do not see the internet as the way forward.

God be with you

Kingsley

Tue 11 Aug

Subject: LMA random heading

Dear Friends

A couple of things before I start. New people, check out eastlandsker.com . Do I have permission from the LMA for Munachlogddu to begin to hold services, and Cyffig in a couple of weeks?

This has been an interesting pilgrimage, some of you have been with me from the very beginning and we started out a relatively small band. So many more have joined us along the way. I have enjoyed your responses, the internet is a two way medium. Yet it is not the same as if we had been physically walking together, there would have been so much more interaction between people. I have enjoyed the two occasions so far when many of us were able to get together, especially the open air service.

As with any pilgrimage this has been an inward journey, perhaps more so because we weren't physically going anywhere, and thanks to your responses and your own stories we have learned from each other. I left a few breadcrumbs along the way about me (6 May, 13 May, 8 June, 29 June, 24 July, 4 August). The journey isn't over yet and I don't know if we will realise we have arrived if we ever do. So for now we step into the future with joy and hope with God as our guide, the best is yet to come.

Walk on

Kingsley

Wed 12 Aug

Subject: haphazard title

Dear Friends

As things slowly open up again it seems so much more difficult to find peace. Yet we need peace more than ever now. We need to find God in the quiet while our lives become busier. As I type this every morning I still find a certain peace and it gives me a chance to reflect. Sometimes I can be sitting here for ages before I can even start and that is quite relaxing too. And I can look out across the valley and think of all the people who have been here, the Mesolithic hunter gatherers, the Neolithic farmers, the Bronze Age warriors, the Iron Age Celts, the pesky Romans, the marauding Irish, the gentle Cistercians, etc. This has been home to so many people and the land has been here for them, it is here for us now and will be here for those who follow after.

We must not be guilty when we do nothing, as long as we don't do it all the time, we owe it to ourselves and to those around us to stop and reflect and simply be. Take a moment now and do nothing.

Silence

Kingsley

Thu 13 Aug

Subject: arbitrary label

Dear Friends

We seem to have drifted into a new normal, we see signs about catching sneezes, signs about 2m distancing, marks on shop floors and on pavements outside, hand sanitizers everywhere, people with masks and it is our way of life now. Imagine if you had been dropped into this suddenly from last year! How quickly we used to things so we hardly notice them any more. But this is life and it is the way we as human beings cope. We adapt and we get on with things even though the world has changed radically. So the question about when things will be back to normal is irrelevant, normal is now. As the joke says, nostalgia isn't what it used to be.

We learn lessons from the past but we live in the present so we must find the joy and happiness today rather than yearn from something that has gone. And there is plenty to look forward to. I know there is still sadness, people lose loved ones, people lose livelihood, the confusion over imposed exam results which will affect so many futures, but human beings are resilient and we will live. There is the image of God in all of us, the spark of the divine, we are all more than we can know, we are all special.

Every blessing

Kingsley

Fri 14 Aug

Subject: LMA unspecific epithet

Dear Friends

We know that God is everywhere and you can talk to him wherever, we also know that the church is not the buildings but the people but sadly not everyone does know this. This is part of the reason why our church buildings are so important, they are a statement to the world. Sadly when the churches were closed I wonder what message was this sending out.

From the beginning the disciples met in the temple which was a sacred place for the Jews, then the upper room became a sacred place after the last supper and they met there as well. As churches were set up in different towns someone with a large enough house set aside a room that became their sacred place, a room they didn't use for anything else not their kitchen or dining room. The Celtic church found places to build wooden buildings that were already sacred, thin places. Not all churches now are in thin places and not all thin places have churches built in them but the church buildings are important wherever they are. They are a physical presence that everyone can recognise, a beacon in an often dark world.

If I had my way all the churches would be open but sadly this is impractical because the rules of the Church in Wales which it has negotiated with the Welsh Assembly are like so many hoops to jump through it is asking a lot for small and often elderly congregations.

We will get there, it may be slow and difficult but nothing worth doing is ever easy. In the meantime we are all salt and light in the world and though at times it seems we cannot change the world who we are will shine through.

Let your little light shine

Kingsley

Sat 15 Aug

Subject: LMA chance rubric

Dear Friends

Another day. Another day for sadness and joy, for tears and laughter, for fear and courage. We human being don't just go through the process of life but live on the rollercoaster of emotions. Sometimes we feel it would be easier to live without them and other times we know we couldn't do without them. We are not ants or bees. We have the ability to dream and to hope and even when our dreams are thwarted or our hopes dashed we can dream and hope again. Time heals but it doesn't ever wipe out the memories both sad and happy, it reminds us that life goes on and there are joys to come. It may rain now but we know it will be sunny again.

Is this what it is to be made in God's image?

Kingsley

Sun 16 Aug

Subject: LMA Trinity 10

Dear Friends

Matt 15:21-28. A Canaanite woman follows Jesus around asking him to heal her daughter and Jesus ignores her, the disciples tell him to send her away so he tells her he only came for Israel, she knelt before him and begged and he said it wasn't right to take the children's bread and toss it to the dogs at which she says the dogs can eat the crumbs that fall from the table. Now he commends her for her faith and her daughter is healed. I am not going to pretend I understand this, I am sure I can look up Bible commentaries and some of you might send me a long sermon explaining it which I won't read because this, like many passages you need to work out for yourself. I, like many of you, do not have all the answers. Is the story about persistence, faith, desperation? Maybe but Jesus' attitude is a mystery. The story certainly doesn't help with the problem of unanswered prayer since I am sure many of you have been just as persistent and still not had an answer.

But those of you who have been following me all the way through will know that despite not having all the answers, despite not understanding a lot of things, I know that God is with us and simple trust is all we can do, that and do our best for one another. Continue to dream and to hope and live and experience joy and love.

Kingsley

Mon 17 Aug

Subject: LMA week 21

Dear Friends

I have always been fascinated by legends and mythology and I often wonder how much they are based on a real event or a story to try to explain something. I also like to think there is mystery in the world and it is not as ordered as some people like to thing. Some people like to explain the miracles of Jesus in practical terms on the assumption that people in his day were dull compared to our modern enlightened selves and were easily impressed. People were never stupid, if we were to try to invent the wheel now we would have to have a committee and we would never agree what colour it should be. When five thousand people gathered to listen to Jesus they didn't know this was going to happen and they would not all have packed bread and fish that morning on the off chance Jesus would be in the area.

Sometimes I do not want an explanation. But I am also a contradiction because I don't take things on face value, I will question. I am restless and always want to know more and perhaps this is at the heart of why I like the idea we can never know everything because it means my wanting to know will never be satisfied. The world is a place of endless wonder and I will never stop looking at it with child-like eyes.

Find something new today

Kingsley

Tue 18 Aug

Subject: LMA

Dear Friends

In a changing world it is comforting to know there are some things that are always there even if we don't always notice them. When I was young I was allowed to stay up late one night to watch the Moon landing and I was excited, this was an amazing event. Strangely enough I have become one of those people who doubt it happened now and I wonder if it is because as I get older I like there to be mysteries as a result of something that happened to me shortly after that affected me in a more profound way.

The Moon is mysterious, it affects us all in a deep way we are not always aware of. Have you noticed how many songs have the Moon popping up unexpectedly even when they are not about the Moon, such as Slow Boat to China, I'll Be Seeing You, A Nightingale Sang in Berkley Square. Apparently a lot of the reason there can be life on this planet is because of the Moon. Ancient people were fascinated by the Moon and attached all sorts of stories and legends to her. The Moon is an ever present part of our lives, and even makes some of our darkest nights light.

The Moon is just one of the many gifts God has given to add stability through uncertain times. Like the Moon God is always there whether we see him or not, he is part of our lives even when we do not acknowledge him. And God has given us so many other things the subject could keep me going until Christmas and beyond.

God is with you

Kingsley

Wed 19 Aug

Subject: LMA

Dear Fiends

I am always amazed at the complexity of us human beings. When reading books we have the ability to be there, to feel the feelings of the characters, even to cry at something sad in the book. Have you noticed that if a favourite book is turned into film it is never as good as our imagined version. If there is no God and we are simply highly evolved animals then what purpose does an imagination like ours possibly serve in the survival of the fittest? With all the other qualities we have our imagination adds extra colour to our lives after all God wants us to have joy. With all the sad things that happen in life, the loss and suffering we need happiness and joy too.

There is so much beauty in this world too. Do you know how many sparrows can fit on a bird table (8" square with a roof)? Eleven. Have you noticed that their markings are all different? When you can't cut the lawn because it is raining have you seen all the different wild flowers that grow in it? Have you noticed how even on a miserable day like today the droplets of water on the blades of grass sparkle like diamonds? It is said 'beauty is in the eye of the beholder' and we have been given eyes to see it and minds to appreciate it if we take time to look for it.

See beauty today.

Kingsley

Thu 20 Aug

Subject: Reflections (from this point I drop the LMA from the subjects because this is no longer simply a LMA email, also they are all called reflections except Sundays and Mondays so I will no longer include them in the book.)

Dear Friends

I have referred to these emails as a pilgrimage we are taking together that started with about twenty pilgrims and has become nearly sixty that I send to directly plus all the people some of you send on to, you are scattered all over the country and in many places in the world too. A pilgrimage is many things, such as a time of fellowship which thanks to your responses we have had a lot of, a time of reflection, a time of sharing, an inner journey to find ourselves to find quiet and to hear God in the silence. But the one thing this pilgrimage is not is a physical journey to a known end. It is still a journey but the end is unknown and I only hope we know we have arrived when we get there.

On a physical journey there is so much to see as the scenery changes, there are often wonderful sights to behold. I haven't travelled much abroad, much preferring wild remote places like the Outer Hebrides and Shetland etc. Part of our journey is always to marvel at the wonderful world we live in and see the hand of God in the awe and majesty of nature as well as in the small and delicate snowdrop. To see God in each other if only we allow God to shine through rather than our selfish selves. To look for good in ourselves and be willing to show this good in our lives.

Kingsley

Fri 21 Aug

Dear Friends

Clunderwen and Llandysilio were added to the parish in 2003, that means I have known P- and A- for 17 years. So when P- asked me to take A-'s funeral I knew I would find it emotional, and when Brighteyes was played as we entered the Crem I almost cried, I hope it never becomes easy. The service was relayed to Nant-Y-Ffin because the Crem can only hold 12 at the moment, and when I got there after the funeral was another emotional moment. To meet up with many of the Clunderwen and Llandysilio people after so long was wonderful. But it was obvious that this lockdown had affected everyone and although it is by no means over each slight easing, each step forward, is a blessing.

We are all seeing the world with different eyes now, we know we cannot take anything for granted. Little things mean so much more now. Though there is sadness, mourning, fear, there are also times for joy. We live with the ups and downs because we are human and we feel. Although the storm is blowing the sun is in the sky above the clouds and it will break through again.

Live every moment.

Kingsley

Sat 22 Aug

Dear Friends

With all the steps forward we have taken, with some of the churches opening, gradually catching up with people again, it is a long way from the early lockdown and yet there is one thing I still haven't been able to do that I miss. I cannot go into someone's house for a cup of tea and have a nice cosy chat. I remember when I was first ordained and was serving my curacy in Llanelli, the Vicar gave me the electoral roll, marked all the regular church goers and told me to visit them. After a few months I surprised him by saying I had visited all them, what do I do now? So he told me to visit everyone else. I wasn't universally welcomed in (Llanelli isn't like round here) but where I was welcome I always found it a privilege, a black shirt and clerical collar can be quite useful. And I find it hard that at the moment I cannot do this.

The Celts understood that every shared meal was in a spiritual sense a reflection of the communion, so even a cup of tea and a piece of cake is sharing with someone on a deep level. Even though we are having services in Church to share communion is such a difficult thing to arrange and until we can share the cup I don't feel we can go that far yet. However through the wonders of the internet we have been sharing on a deep and spiritual level all through this strange time, and even Jesus found that talking to the woman at the well and changing her life satisfied his physical hunger. Communion is an outward and physical sign of a spiritual truth and if we

19

are in Jesus and he in us it is enough. And we look forward to the time when we can share food and drink again.

Kingsley

Sun 23 Aug

Subject: Trinity 11

Dear Friends

Matthew 16:13-20. This is an interesting passage. Jesus asks his disciples who people say he is and they tell him some of the rumours, John the Baptist, Elijah, Jeremiah, etc. which is interesting in itself as the Jews didn't believe in reincarnation. But Jesus was leading up to his next question which was to ask directly who they thought he was. Simon Peter immediately said he was the Messiah, the Son of God. Then Jesus made Peter the rock on which the church was built which even the gates of hell could not prevail against.

Too often we repeat what other people say rather that what we think, or we say the things we want others to hear either to impress or more often just to fit in. Faced with a direct question about our own thoughts or beliefs would we have the courage of Peter just to say what we really believed? Over the course of these emails it is interesting who responds to what, you are such a wide range of different individuals and there is no way I can write something that will please everyone nor will everyone agree. When we only mix with people who have the same basic beliefs as ourselves we get to think we are always right. The challenge is to mix with people with different views, to admit we can be wrong or that our way of looking at something is not the only way, but be willing to say what we really believe and be true to ourselves.

The rock on which the church is built is the courage to speak out, pity it lost its way.

Kingsley

Part 2
Opening Up

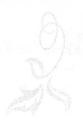

Mon 24 Aug

Subject: Week 22

Dear Friends

Firstly can I ask permission of the LMA to open St David's, Clunderwen. And tell all the new people about eastlandsker.com which is always worth a look in case I have updated it.

It was good to see so many people at St Mary's yesterday, sorry if I was a bit brief only after all these emails I am running out of new things to say! I hope everything went well in Mynachlogddu as well.

Talking of Mynachlogddu, St Dogmael was obviously a local saint, I didn't come across him when I did my dissertation (aka A Celtic Parish) so don't know much about him, nor did I come across St Brynach (Llanboidy) because I only had four churches at the time as well as a scattering of closed churches. I found the dedication of churches quite interesting, Mary never came to Whitland, David never came to Clunderwen, there is some doubt that Tysilio came to Llandysilio, there was no Saint Mallteg and as for Cyffig! Cyffig has no dedication because a Kyffig was a Norse word for cell or small place, in other words a Viking became a Christian and settled in a small stone hut there as a hermit. Hermits were reckoned to be wise people who others would go to see for insight, I wonder how they thought of something new to say every day for years.

But St Canna did found Llangan, she was related to many of the well know Welsh saints, she also went to Cardiff - Pont Cana, Canton (Cannas Town). This was an age of hermits and saints, they were closer to God and miracles happened because miracles were simply part of life. When we believe simply things will happen, we will not need to make a song and dance about it.

Simply believe.

Kingsley

Tue 25 Aug

Dear Friends

As I visit some of my churches with the aim of opening them again I have to be cautious, is it what I want or is it what the congregations want and each time the response is that it is what they want. One of the functions of the church that has tended to be overlooked is the social getting together which is not the same online. We can pray anywhere, we can find God anywhere but we cannot find each other anywhere. I will admit I found the full lockdown refreshing, it gave me a chance to take things easier and to reflect, to find God and to find myself again. But I did not get into this job to sit on my behind and meditate, God managed to push me into it because I wanted to help people and although from your responses to these emails I have been able to do this to a certain extent I actually need to be out there with you.

One of my great joys at the moment is St Mary's and how important it is for people to have a church to come to, though we are pushing the present capacity of the church under the social distancing regulations. To be able to come together and celebrate being able to worship collectively, to look for joy and hope with one another and to seek the common good. The lockdown took a great toll on us all and it has not gone away but as we slowly emerge we find strength in each other, look for the positive and give thanks.

Abundant blessings

Kingsley

Wed 26 Aug

Dear Friends

There are so many frightening reports floating around, the second wave, food shortages and such like. We are not out of this yet but we still cannot predict the future. The pandemic is still largely an unknown and perhaps it is wise to prepare for the worst. But at the beginning of all this large temporary hospitals were built and barely used, the NHS coped though it was hard pressed. I know I am an optimist and perhaps I do tend to see things too positively but I honestly do not believe things are ever as dark as they are painted and I have found this throughout my life.

Whatever the future holds now is a time to grab joy and happiness where we can and if there are troubles ahead they too will pass. When Pandora opened the box and let out all the evils into the world there was still hope in the bottom, legend though this is it is obviously an observation of how things are. And the hope that God gives is no legend it is a promise.

I wish you joy today

Kingsley

Thu 27 Aug

Dear Friends

As we meet up with more people we haven't seen for a long time because of the lockdown do we notice a change in them? This has been a big thing in all of our lives and it has affected us all in different ways and none of us can be exactly the same as before.

From an early age how much are we truly ourselves and how much are we fulfilling other people's expectations of us? Or, even more complicated, our belief of what others expect of us? During the lockdown we were forced to be ourselves with no expectations from anyone else and if we have learned anything about ourselves I hope we can continue to be more true to who we are. Because the person we are is the person God wanted us to be not what others want us to be. I hope this does not make us more selfish because human beings are supposed to be social creatures, and one of the most important of Jesus' teachings is how we can help one another. In 'The Neverending Story' there is a mirror that reveals your true self and very few people can face this, but I hope the magic mirror of the lockdown has revealed something to ourselves that we like and we can carry into our new future. I also hope it has helped us realise we need space for ourselves in an increasingly busy life and we will not fill our time with unnecessary things.

Take time to reflect today

Kingsley

Fri 28 Aug

Dear Friends

There are two parts of what is known as the butterfly affect, one is about time travel and the repercussions of going back into the remote past and accidentally stepping on a butterfly and changing history, something we don't have to worry about. The other is a butterfly flaps its wings and a storm happens the other side of the world, this can't be measured or even validated but the idea is that this world is such a complicated system the least little movement somehow has consequences for the whole. Then you can go into quantum physics where every sub atomic particle affects every other sub atomic particle in some way. But these emails are not about quasi science or quantum physics but about people.

As we live in this life we are a part of the whole, every action we make has consequences. Shout at someone in the morning and they are grumpy to everyone they meet who in turn are grumpy to everyone else. Smile and joke with someone in the morning and they smile to everyone they meet and so on. Our whole life affects so many people in so many ways we can have no idea of our value to humanity as a whole, no wonder John Donne wrote 'No man is an island ...' Every life counts, none of us are simply a statistic, every death affects us all. Our faith as Christians affects the overall goodness of the world without having to shout about it or condemn the world as evil. The little kindnesses we do will have an impact even when we don't know it. Don't expect to know how we have helped other people, simply spread kindness and joy wherever we go.

Kingsley

Sat 29 Aug

Dear Friends

It is a good time for the amateur astronomer, the Moon, Jupiter and Saturn are in the same area of sky, if only we had a clear sky. Did you know that moon starer is an anagram of astronomer? There is nothing like looking up into the night sky and looking at the stars and the planets, it gives you a bit of perspective when you contemplate the vastness of space, how small and insignificant we actually are. If the universe is there simply as a random consequence of an enormous explosion then we are meaningless. And yet we know in our inner beings that we are not, why do we feel we have importance if this is all one big accident? Surely even the most ardent of atheists cannot explain that. If there is no God there is no meaning. But God who created the vastness of the universe, the Maker Of All Things, knows us all by name and has even numbered the hairs on our heads, he knows us better than we know ourselves and will take us to himself when our time here is over.

And in the meantime he has designed the most beautiful of worlds, if only we didn't try to spoil it, for us to appreciate beauty and find happiness and joy. He has given us minds to explore and learn new things all the time, he has given us hearts to love but they are so delicate they can break. He has given us art and words and music, he has given us his likeness so we can create. Why waste all that on being bitter and greedy and envious and nasty. Appreciate what you have and live your life to the full.

Kingsley

Sun 30 Aug

Subject: Trinity 12

Dear Friends

Matthew 16.21-28. Jesus is leading his disciples onward to Jerusalem and warns them that he must die and be raised to life again, Peter tries to stop him and gets rebuked and they are all warned about the dangers and told of the rewards of following him. Jesus came to do many things but central to his purpose was to die for us and so our future is safe in his hands, therefore it is not about the next life that we should be thinking but how we live in this one (see also Romans 12.9-21 the NT reading for today), we are asked to repay good for evil, to do our best to live at peace with everyone.

Some people do make it hard to live at peace with, they look for fault, they throw your smile back at you with a scowl. We cannot change others if they want to be like that, all we are asked is that we do our best to be loving and kind. I know it is hard at times but bitterness and jealousy and hatred can eat away at you so it is always best not to go there in the first place but have joy and love in your heart no matter what others are like. And if you can keep that bright spark within your heart it will carry you through all the dark times in life and give you hope for the future.

Kingsley

Mon 31 Aug

Subject: week 23

Dear Friends

One of my greatest joys yesterday was to see so many in St Mary's, though not for my sake but for those who came, for those who feel they need to come together for worship and fellowship (and a chat). Gradually people are having the courage to spread their wings. It is only a simple service, with no hymns, and I would not be comfortable with a communion service, and I cannot go up into the pulpit, and it is barely half an hour, and we are pushing the bounds of the present seating capacity. And people still come, because although we all know God is everywhere there is still something special about setting aside a time on a Sunday to actually go to a church, it is part of our discipline. It also gives us some structure to our week although I still find it difficult trying to work out which day I am in the rest of the week.

I have often commented in these reflections about the sense of presence in the church, I have said there is an angel but it is also the centuries of prayer. Although we are bound in time God is not and from his perspective we are all there stretching back through history and on into the future, all together offering him worship and prayer, we are part of the great crowd of witnesses. Each of us individually add to the overall goodness and light in the world and when we gather together the power of that light is magnified like a beacon on a hill. And as more churches open the light of the beacon is spread to other hills and a message is sent across the land. And the rest of the week we continue to carry the light into the community.

Shine on.

Kingsley

Tue 1 Sept

Dear Friends

Some symbolism is so old no one knows when it began. In Celtic art there is the Celtic knot, a thread that weaves within itself that has no beginning and no end and there is the snake or dragon that twists round itself and bites its own tail, but these symbols are possibly older than the Celts although no one really knows how far back the Celts go anyway. In any case the knot symbolises eternity and the snake or dragon symbolises life death and rebirth. Both are ways of showing what the ancient people understood about continuity and about the cycle of life, the seasons, the very universe itself.

Some people would argue that Christianity adopted these symbols and overlaid its own message on them. But it is all part of the natural world that God has made, he has put into the very fabric of existence signs that point to him, and Jesus was the ultimate revelation of this and he brought all the strands together. He showed in his own life, death and resurrection what this all means.

Too many people live in a technological, throw away age and no longer see this. While those who are closer to the soil understand it. In the same way those who seek power and importance no longer understand people, yet it is people who are the world, who are the church and keep everything going.

Kingsley

Wed 2 Sept

Dear Friends

At the beginning of the lockdown I was on an inner journey which may have come across in my earlier emails and I learned a lot about myself. The danger now as things get busier, such as Cyffig and Clunderwen opening on 13th and the Bishop coming to Cyffig on 27th, is that I forget what I have learned. I do find this time when I sit at the computer and sometimes sit for 15 minutes before I start typing it is a chance to find that inner peace. When St Mary's first opened for private prayer that was a good time just to sit and not even think at times, to feel the presence that is in the church, now we have services we fill the space with words, I wonder how long a church full of people can sit quietly with nothing said without someone wondering when we are going to start.

A river flowing down from the hills has its periods of waterfalls and rapids, it has its places where it rushes in full flow, but there are places where it calmly meanders and is at peace, but it will always reach the sea. There is nothing wrong with taking time out of busy lives just to drift, we will get there in the end.

Take a moment to do nothing

Kingsley

Thu 3 Sept

Dear Friends

A lot of people recently have been commenting on the way things are, although we are able to get about more and do more we cannot do things casually as we once could but have to think about everything, assess the risks in our minds, be aware of social distancing and so forth. The schools having started back I wonder how the teachers and the children are managing with the new ways, but they are able to meet up with friends again and start to think about their futures again and interact again like they could not through the internet. I, on the other hand, have got a lot of zoom meetings with the church coming up! Enough said.

God so loved the world that he didn't send a text.

I am pleased that the Bishop is coming to Cyffig, unfortunately the present capacity is 14, that means Deb's family and friends, the small Cyffig congregation, the Bishop and no more. The original plan for the confirmation back in April was for there to be no other services in the parish group and everyone to come to Cyffig, but we cannot do this now. But at least the Confirmation can go ahead so please pray for Deb on 27th even though you can't be there in person.

On our journey we have come over a rise in the ground but we are not there yet, there is still a way to go but we have come a long way since March.

Safe journey

Kingsley

Fri 4 Sept

Dear Friends

The old Vicarage was secluded, in off the road, surrounded by trees. When this new one was built they cut down most of the trees and built almost on the roman road so the front is very open, and everyone walking along can look up into it. At the beginning of the lockdown everyone seemed to be walking by, now there are fewer and they have got used to Y Ficerdy and aren't staring at it all the time. Today the children from Dyffryn Taf have started their cross country run (or walk) past here. A large group walked by just now, chatting and laughing and it was good to see such normality. Whatever the risks children need to learn and a lot of their learning is from each other.

Human beings are not meant to be solitary. I will admit it is good to get away at times but I would soon miss company. I have often said being a Vicar is a good job for a nosey person, apart from the awkward and nasty few I find people fascinating. Everyone has their own story, their own point of view, their own joys and sorrows, their children they are proud of, their own interests. Older people can teach us wisdom, younger people can remind us of our youth. Everyone is important, they have their own place in the rich tapestry of the world. I would hate it if I only mixed with people who were the same as me or always agreed with me. Our differences, our uniqueness is vital to stop us being too self-engrossed.

Learn something new from someone today

Kingsley

Sat 5 Sept

Dear Friends

Each time I go into one of the churches of the group for the first time in ages I find it an emotional experience. Yesterday it was St Brynach's, Llanboidy. I had a burial of ashes so I arranged to meet everyone after the short service to discuss opening the church again for services. (Is everyone in the LMA in favour?). I got there before the burial and went into the church which I found moving, and I had to say hello to Grief who must have been feeling very lonely (Google the church to understand this). More than this, it was good to see people I have not seen for a long time - welcome to these musings those of you I now have email addresses for, check out eastlandsker.com. Of my five churches this only leaves St Tysilio, which I must sort out soon.

So the earth rolls onward into the future, each day is a new opportunity, each day brings its sorrows and its joys, each day brings worries but above all brings hope. Day follows night, seasons come and go, the journey continues, make the most of every moment and look forward to a brighter future.

I wish you peace

Kingsley

Sun 6 Sept

Subject: Trinity 13

Dear Friends

Romans 13:8-14. I always thought Paul was one of the religious elite in Jewish circles but in this passage he mentions four of the more obvious commandments then says 'and whatever other commandments there may be,' so I don't feel so bad that I can never remember all ten. However, Paul is merely writing to the Jews in Rome what Jesus had said, that love is the fulfilment of the law and the only thing we should owe one another is love. Always a hard thing to do considering some of the people we come across! He also tells to wake up, face the light of day and put the acts of darkness behind us, for light itself is our armour.

In light there is no darkness, in the light nothing can be hidden. For Christians living in the light is the only way, to be open and honest and loving no matter what other people are like. Living in this world it doesn't always seem possible but light is our best weapon against the evils that surround us. Living in the light we have no fear. Soon it is the equinox and after that the nights become longer than the days, but Jesus came on the darkest of days to be a light in the world. Let us be lights in this world too.

Kingsley

Mon 7 Sept

Subject: week 24

Dear Friends

We walk a narrow line. As I press ahead with opening churches it is good to see so many turn up because they want to, but there is still a lot of concern because although the death rate for COVID-19 is very low the number of cases is going up and people are afraid of a second wave. On the other hand there are those who resent the current restrictions and don't believe they are necessary, but I was talking to a neighbour yesterday whose best mate died of the virus.

So we continue to walk this narrow line and as we take forward steps we take them sensibly and with great thought and preparation. This is the present normal.

And yet, I saw so much joy in people yesterday, so much thankfulness, so much sharing, so much hope. For all that is negative there is so much more good. You will find the strength within yourself, there is tremendous power in the human heart, and the hand of God is there to lead you.

Walk in the light

Kingsley

Tue 8 Sept

Dear Friends

Time is one of those mysteries I will never understand. Looking back at some of my earlier emails I was finding April was such a long month, it was going on for ever and by May I felt it ought to be September. But now it is September and somewhere the time has disappeared. I have often commented on age but what is that? Only the number of times the earth has gone round the sun while we have been sitting on it. From our perspective we have a finite amount of it on this earth though an infinity before us afterwards, which we cannot begin to comprehend. Imagine what time is like for the spiritual beings like angels, they can have no comprehension of it at all.

Time is invisible and apart from breaking down the cycle of the seasons and the days into smaller pieces which clocks count away we cannot really measure it. It goes and it cannot be replaced. Time not spent with someone cannot be remade. Opportunities not taken cannot be retaken. Time is like a thief we cannot see or stop. Time not spent well will fill us with regret. And yet time needs to be given to peace and reflection and not just filled with things. The time we have needs to be enjoyed and not wished away. Even when we wait we must make the most of that time too. The time I spend with you all through this medium I value so much I don't ever want to stop, it calms me before the day and makes me think.

Appreciate time today.

Kingsley

Wed 9 Sept

Dear Friends

A Celtic Blessing I am using every Sunday:

May the road rise up to meet you.

May the wind be always at your back.

May the sun shine warm upon your face;

the rains fall soft upon your fields

and until we meet again,

may God hold you in the palm of His hand.

The Celts understand the interconnectedness of everything, God, nature and us. They don't compartmentalise things, you could say they have a holistic approach to the whole of life. Many of the troubles of modern life is that we tend to do the opposite, we break our lives into sections and very often it is our spiritual welfare that gets put into a box and tucked away as unimportant. Another danger of this is that we don't see ourselves as part of humanity as a whole. Yet if the lockdown taught us anything it is that we need each other, in helping others we are helped ourselves, and as we meet up with people again it brings great joy. Another impression I get from the Celtic Church with its holistic approach was that the distinction between clergy and laity was very blurred, and with fewer clergy and our reliance more and more on the laity I hope this is the case now, we are one people. The days of one church one Vicar and the Vicar did everything has gone and it was not a golden age that we miss. Everyone is vital to the life of the church.

Kingsley

Part 3
Second Wave

Thu 10 Sept

Dear Friends

A second wave, local lockdowns, stricter restrictions, it is worrying and I know a lot of people are worried. And yet there are fewer deaths now for many reasons, nor was the original threat anywhere as bad is it was forecast, 500,000 people did not die in the UK and the big new hospitals that were built were barely used if at all. We must all be sensible but not afraid.

Fear is the devil's weapon which is why I will never be afraid and I will continue to try and give comfort and hope. 1 Corinthians 13:13 'And now these three remain: faith, hope and love. But the greatest of these is love.' Faith at times is very difficult to cling on to with some of the things we have to face in life but cling on we must. Hope seems an insipid thing when we say at times 'I hope so' but hope is actually a promise and a guarantee and will take away despair. And as for love, love is our most powerful emotion, it is what binds us together. Without love we are selfish and unkind and separated from others. With it we can face anything even loss and heartbreak because love transcends this world, through the thin veil that separates us from those we have lost love is still a bond with them that cannot be broken. And I do not mean contacting the dead or hearing messages but knowing in our hearts that we are not that far apart and will meet again and it is only time in between and time is nothing. Jesus defeated death, what is there left to fear? Therefore do not fear but have faith, hope and love.

Believe

Kingsley

Fri 11 Sept

Dear Friends

This daily message is a two way street and I am grateful to all of you who take the time to reply. I am also humbled by some of your responses, people who face difficult situations and yet find my ramblings helpful. But if we cannot reach out to help or give comfort even in a small way what is our purpose. I hear so many stories of good and caring people, unsung heroes, and these are the backbone of humanity, these are the people who make the world a wonderful place. For all the bad that is reported in the news there is a vast amount more good, and this gives us faith, hope and love.

Every so often someone will ask how I manage to write this every day, well this is not just me, I respond to things people say, their concerns. This is a conversation between me and you. It also helps to be widely read, willing to listen, have an IQ the same as Einstein (so much for humble), as well as being a dreamer and rather strange. But mostly this is not about me it is about all of you and I cannot get over how this has taken off. You are the salt and light in the world, you make the difference.

Humbly yours

Kingsley

Sat 12 Sept

Dear Friends

So this is the second wave. Some restrictions have been imposed. Yet this is a precaution, there are still fewer deaths from the virus, and none in Wales for well over a week. So as Corporal Jones would say 'Don't panic', which by a strange coincidence are the words of the cover of 'The Hitchhikers Guide to the Galaxy' in large friendly letters.

I am not your self-appointed bringer of good cheer, I volunteered. You may remember I initially turned down the offer of LMA Dean, I remember the good old days when meetings took place in rooms, I attended a meeting of the new (and proposed) LMA Deans in the boardroom at the Diocesan Office where I stated in front of everyone that it was not possible to form a Local Ministry Area of fifteen churches from Clydau to Pendine with only two full time clergy. Then, because of the rumours of the parishes being split up and put in different LMA's both of us full time clergy went to a meeting in Haverfordwest about the LMA's in the hopes of finding out what was going on. The Archdeacon chatted to us over lunch, he agreed the proposed LMA needed three full time clergy and promised there would be a third, but one of us would have to be LMA Dean. So I volunteered and the Bishop went out of her way to thank me. The LMA was inaugurated in St Mary's then WHAM! COVID-19 and lockdown.

Two days later I sent my first circular email just to show I was still here and if anyone needed me here I was. So I repeat what I said then, 'Hello from your friendly LMA Dean', and I am still here.

But this is not complete lockdown this time. The Church of England has checked with the Government and places of worship can stay open and more than six people can gather for services of worship, I hope the Church in Wales follows suit and I will let you know as soon as I hear anything. And a quick word about face masks in shops - 'MMMMMph mumble mumble.'

Keep the faith, love and hope.

Kingsley

Sun 13 Sept
Subject: Trinity 14

Dear Friends

Romans 14:1-12. This is the passage where Paul talks about accepting people with different levels of faith and different ways of expressing it without judging because

Christ died for all. Yet you will always find people who have decided at what level a person is a Christian and below this they are not. As a Vicar if someone comes to me to christen their baby I accept that for whatever reason they have come to the church for something they don't need to do therefore there must be some spark of faith somewhere. Some would say it is only for the party after and grumble that they are only using the church but people don't need an excuse for a party and how can we possibly know what is in someone else's mind.

We cannot judge someone else's faith because they do not believe the same as me. I know people who do this and I expect I don't measure up to what they would require. The message is that we do not have to reach a certain level to be loved and accepted by God. We do not have to fill in a form and tick certain boxes except 'Did Christ die for me?' Yes. Despite the number of times in the Bible we are told not to judge people still do. Do not let anyone judge you for your level of faith or your beliefs, only you know your own heart and mind. John 14:2 'In my Father's house are many rooms; if it were not so, I would have told you. I am going there to prepare a place for you.'

Kingsley

Mon 14 Sept

Subject: week 25

Dear Friends

St David's, Clunderwen had its first service yesterday thanks to Nathan but I haven't heard how it went yet.

Cyffig also had its first service and it was good to be there again and for the small congregation to meet up. Today there is the six people rule (churches being exempt) and masks in shops, I haven't been into a shop yet! Plusses and minuses, I suppose this is what we can expect at the moment with the worrying increase in infections though not deaths. We cannot drift through life but have to think what we are doing all the time and be ready for changes in the rules.

On a different note, I have been watching the birds on the pile of cut branches queueing up for the bird table. One of the sparrows is always dressed for the occasion wearing his bow tie (yes a dickie bow), and his name is Bird, James Bird. We see shapes in all sorts of things and our imaginative minds see things such as castles in the clouds, Jesus in tea leaves, smiley faces in cucumbers, cats that look like Hitler. Have you wondered why we do this? It is not something we choose to do it is just natural. Perhaps it is our minds trying to make sense of things around us or add a bit of mystery to ordinary objects, whatever it is it is another incredible part of who we are, another gift from God. Appreciate your imagination today.

Kingsley

Tue 15 Sept

Dear Friends

Sad news, the wearing of face masks in church is mandatory, but at least we can still hold services and are not limited to six.

I have always liked autumn, there is a calm about it somehow. Often at this time of year a mist settles in the valley that is reminiscent of the lake that was here after the last ice age. The leaves of the trees begin to turn from green to varying shades of red and orange and yellow before falling to the ground where they can be blown into heaps that children can run through and kick into the air. The air itself has an edge to it especially in the early morning. The fruit trees are laden with fruit and those annoying brambles try to make up for it by providing countless berries. I have always liked harvest in church, to open the door and smell the flowers and the produce that people have taken time to provide and arrange.

Because of the lockdown the church year has not been such a driving force and I wonder how many of the celebrations to come we can do, surely we can but on a smaller scale. Without Easter, Ascension, Pentecost, Trinity I for one have been more able to reflect on how these events were for the Disciples rather than for us. This time has given me the space to reflect on what is important and what really the church is about. As we have been able to come together for worship again it stands out that it is the gathering together of people that is important rather than the form of worship and this we will continue to do.

Appreciate today.

Kingsley

Wed 16 Sept

Dear Friends

St Peter's, Lampeter Velfrey are holding an open air harvest service this Sunday, I trust this is OK with the LMA. I am going to see the folk at St Tysilio's, Llandysilio on Friday, do I have the LMA's permission to open that church for regular services? I am also going to Clydey on Saturday but I think I already asked about that. Slowly, bit by bit, the church is opening up again. It is interesting that places of worship have been given exemption to the six people rule and I wonder have the powers that be woken up to the fact that the churches are important to the people after the huge outcry at closing the churches at the beginning of the lockdown.

It is a glorious autumn day, the mist has slowly cleared and the dew bejewelled spider webs are spread across lawns and hedges, the sun is shining brightly in the sky. Today I will be preparing for Sunday as it is the only day I have spare this week yet despite being busy I still take time to reflect, to reach out to God, to chat to people I meet down in Whitland, I have learned something from the complete lockdown earlier this year and that is to give myself space. I enjoy this time now as I sit and look at the view and ramble away on the keyboard (this is the third rewrite today) so I ask all of you to take time today to do nothing, appreciate what is around you and the people you know and open yourself to God for a moment.

Peace

Kingsley

Thu 17 Sept

Dear Friends

I am sure there were times during the first and second world wars when the people living through them thought the wars would never end, and these went on for years, but they did end. And in both cases the world had changed. This pandemic will end and the world will be a different place. There will always be far reaching consequences but we will live with those as well. We cope, we adapt, we learn, we grow, we live on and there are plenty of joys to come. During the wars songwriters wrote songs of hope, why has no one now? Why so much doom and gloom? We all need encouragement, we need some rousing speeches from our leaders, we need the promise of hope.

The church should be setting an example, at least more and more church buildings are open which is a good sign, and our Bishop is coming to Cyffig on the 27th which is a very positive statement, but where is Justin Welby in all this? Still, all of you who read this know where I am, I am only an email away if you need me and I have bucket loads of optimism. I pray for each of you as I type in your email addresses, and I hope those of you who send this on pray for everyone on your lists.

Put your hand in the hand of Jesus and let him lead you through these worrying times.

Kingsley

Fri 18 Sept

Dear Friends

A friend remarked recently that everywhere looks like a crime scene. There are tapes blocking off places, marking the floors, across the pews in church. Well, there has been a major incident and it is still ongoing. I have seen and heard about such a wide range of reactions to this, from the casual carrying on as if nothing has happened to the terrified even of going out. I am trying to take a sensible approach, being careful and abiding by the rules while getting as much back to normality as possible. This is why I am keen to open churches while following the Church in Wales guidelines. I cannot go into people's houses but I can meet them in the garden, our churches are limited for space because of social distancing and we have to wear masks, we cannot sing or cwtch.

And still the earth turns on its axis and continues its path around the sun, autumn has come and nature is carrying on as it always has. The natural cycle of life continues with death and new life, there are still occasions we can celebrate even if only a few of us can gather to do so. There is the confirmation coming up and I will be taking a wedding soon and at least the churches are exempt from the six people rule, though we do have a reduced capacity - St Mary's 25, Cyffig 14 and so on so people can't just casually turn up. I wonder if a smaller gathering for a celebration is somehow more meaningful, more intimate, more personal and more dignified.

One thing I have learned through this major incident and that is to appreciate everything, even the small things, and to make the most of meeting people.

Enjoy today

Kingsley

Sat 19 Sept

Dear Friends

I was in St Tysilio's yesterday and I am on my way to Clydai this afternoon. On Tuesday I am going to St Peter's, Lampeter Velfrey (do they have the LMA's permission to open for services?). In the midst of the second wave it is good to have something positive to report. And I am getting really good at filling in Risk Assessment forms.

I hate forms, I hate filling in boxes but it is necessary at times. I also don't like having everything prepared in detail before I do it. People sometimes ask me what I am going to say in certain situations and I never know, I never plan what I am going to say. I even gave up writing sermons very quickly into my Curacy in Llanelli, the only sermons I prepare are Christmas and Easter and even then only a few notes. I like spontaneity, although certain aspects of my life are quite ordered but I use the order as a framework to work around rather than the box I work within. We cannot predict what is going to happen, how people around us are going to react, who we will meet along the way.

It also doesn't pay to be too rigid in our thinking or our beliefs. It is also OK to doubt and to question God, otherwise when tragedy strikes we have no space to mourn because we expect ourselves not to and we will then feel we are letting God down with our human feelings. Even Jesus on the cross cried out 'My God, my God, why have you forsaken me.' But God had not, nor does he forsake us and when our lives are shattered he will hold the pieces.

Kingsley

Sun 20 Sept

Subject: Trinity 15

Dear Friends

Matthew 20:1-16. This is the parable of the workers in the vineyard, as the day wears on the owner hires more and more people and at the end of the day they are all paid the same wage. Those who worked all day grumbled that they had the same wage as those who came late. From our perspective this seems unfair but you have to realise that in heaven there is no higher or lower position, all are equal, and eternal life is eternal and you cannot have more than that. There is no greater or lesser reward, and it is a gift of God anyway.

If this is the way God sees things, after all he sent his Son to be a servant, why are we so fixated with ranking and levels of importance? Yet so many people are, they strive for the important positions, for prestige, and some who do not have either will gravitate to and fawn over those who have. We live in a culture of celebrity and the media throws stuff about well-known people at us as if we are interested, sadly so many are ready to lap it up. Not being a television watcher I haven't a clue who most of them are. When will we learn that we are all equal in the sight of God, and he is interested in the lives of everyone and the best accolade anyone can get is 'Well done, good and faithful servant, ... Come and share your masters happiness!' (Mt 25:23)

Kingsley

Mon 21 Sept

Subject: Week 26

Dear Friends

We cannot plan our lives minutely because we cannot see what is ahead. We can put things in our diary that we intend to do but we cannot pencil in the unexpected. This is certainly the case at the moment when the rules to cope with the virus change all the time. Even so, this has always been the case. We often wish we knew the future but we have to live a day at a time.

A day at a time. We are not given our whole life in one go, unlike a story in a book where we can skip to the end to see what happens, we have to experience it as it happens. We have to live through the good times and the bad, the happy and the sad, the joys and the worries. Every experience we face becomes part of what forms us into the future, it is part of our personal story that builds into our life. And our lives are woven in and through all those we meet especially those we are close to, and it is often referred to as a rich tapestry. Each life is an important part of everyone else's life, no one is unimportant, value everyone you meet today and make the most of every moment.

Kingsley

Tue 22 Sept

Dear Friends

Today is the equinox, which is Greek for equal night because the length of the day and the night is the same. It also officially marks the beginning of autumn, how fitting then that the recent run of bright sunny days has given way to mist and rain. It is of course a significant day for pre-Christian people and this is because when the middle stone age passed into the new stone age the people were becoming farmers and marking such events were important for planting, growing and harvesting.

St Mary's church as I have said before is built in an elliptical enclosure that would have been what we now call a henge that is aligned with the rising sun of the equinox. Perhaps there would have been some sort of religious rite and a celebration to mark the occasion, and of course this is a harvest festival. However St Mary's have always celebrated harvest on the first Sunday of October and if you want to be a Christian purist then it is still a pagan festival. But so what, so much of when the church does things is based around pre-Christian events because pre-Christian does not mean pre-God. God, the Maker Of All Things has given us signs pointing to himself in the whole of nature and we cannot dismiss the past simply because we in our arrogance think we know better or like to feel superior.

At the beginning of the lockdown we were finding God everywhere, he is in and through everything. If you look closely enough at anything and know what to look for you can find 'Made by God' stamped on it, on the very atoms and sub atomic particles.

Appreciate all that God has made today.

Kingsley

Wed 23 Sept

Dear Friends

Two things before I start. Can I have the LMA's permission to open St David's, Llanddewi Velfry for services and I have updated the website eastlandsker. com.

I know this is going to annoy some of you but I am grateful to Richard Law for 'Eglwys St Clydai a History and Guide' who agrees with me about the Romans, in fact he points out something I hadn't even thought of, by Romanising the Celtic Church meant that money would flow back to Rome. He also mentions something that I had heard yet sadly there is no proof of, that Christianity may have come to this country with Joseph of Arimathaea before the Romans. If all of this is true it does put a totally different slant on Christianity in this country and who knows may point the way ahead, to let go of rigid organisation and put more trust in the local congregations and this is certainly the impression I have been getting ever since I was Area Dean of South Pembrokeshire and now as LMA Dean of East Landsker and meeting up with the people who run their churches. We need structure as a church, even the Celtic Church had a structure, but we need a lot more freedom locally. But I am the sort of person who uses structure to build on and expand outward from rather than a box to work within.

We cannot put God in a box either, we cannot say this is what God does and no further, we cannot say we know everything about God. We cannot catalogue all that God is as the sum total of who he is and what he does. We are living in an age when he is going to do something totally new, in fact I think he has already started and I don't think we can look back at any history as a guide to his new work. The world has already changed and so has the church, and one obvious consequence I have seen as we open more and more churches is that the likes of me have become less important because I cannot go from church to church on a Sunday or visit people in their homes because of the risks, the church has already become a church of everyone with the people taking their own services and communities caring for one another in a far more obvious way. Whether they like it or not Clergy have become less necessary, gone completely is the Victorian idea that the Vicar did everything. So what is my role? Gentle oversight as it says in the Inauguration Service.

Kingsley

Thu 24 Sept

Dear Friends

Not long ago things were beginning to look quite bright and hopeful and now all of a sudden there is doom and gloom everywhere, or so it seems. Six months of this new clampdown seems such a long time. Yet as I have said before both World Wars were longer and with all the devastation and loss of life and livelihood people got through them but people could sing and songwriters were writing songs of hope. Where is the voice of hope and optimism in our present situation, where are the rousing speeches?

This is why I refuse to give in to fear and despondency, someone has to, and I am grateful for all your positive messages back. We are stronger than we think, I have seen this over and over again. It is interesting to note that all over the world different animals live in different habitats, some thrive in heat others in cold, some like it damp and others dry. You will not find penguins in the Sahara or camels in the Antarctic. Yet you will find human beings everywhere. We are incredibly adaptable, we are great survivors, we always find a way. We are, after all, made in God's image which is our intellect, our power to dream, our creativity. Let nothing get you down, or not for long anyway, there is always tomorrow, there is always more to do, more to see, more to learn.

Find something new today.

Kingsley

Fri 25 Sept

Dear Friends

I have heard this year referred to as 'The Lost Year' a few times now. I wonder how history will refer to it? But it is not lost, many things are happening, life has still gone on. Many people have suffered many things, and there is hardship still to come, and there are many positive things to come out of it too. In the early complete lockdown before we knew what was ahead many people took time to reassess their lives, to change what they thought was important and with the churches closed they found God everywhere.

Often in the Bible people are referred to as sheep and you can see why, at the beginning of the lockdown people were panic buying (especially toilet rolls) because everyone else was, the moment restrictions were lifted people flooded the beaches because everyone else did, now they are panic buying again. I know this is a generalisation but it does make me wonder about collective humanity, how crowds could be cheering Jesus one day and jeering him another. Where is individuality?

We need to be willing to stand out and be different, not afraid of the crowds. We need to be true to ourselves and the unique people we are. We need to be leaders and not followers, we need to make a difference.

Make a difference today.

Kingsley

Sat 26 Sept

Dear Friends

As Llanelli goes into lockdown my mind goes back to the four years I spent as a Curate there. I enjoyed my time there and as a Curate you don't have many responsibilities. But in a place like Llanelli because of the size of population I only knew the church people, when I came to Whitland as Vicar I got to know so many local people and not just the church people. When I was in Llanelli people were bemoaning the fact that they had to lock their doors now and couldn't just pop into each other's houses, each area of Llanelli once had been a small community in itself but that had gone. Some people like towns and cities because there is so much more going on but I much prefer smaller communities. In towns and cities you can get lost in a crowd where you can't in places like Whitland. Even before lockdown I had taken to not wearing my collar all the time because people knew who I was anyway.

At the moment it is more obvious that the government treats us as statistics or numbers, but that is the role of governments, to treat us a country as a whole rather than each of us as individuals. It is in our communities that we are individuals, where we are known for who we are, and when people want to know your business it is not out of nosiness (I hope) but interest and concern. And God does not treat us as a world, even with his plans for the world, he knows us all as individuals and we are all special in his eyes.

Kingsley

Sun 27 Sept

Subject: Trinity 16

Dear Friends

Matthew 21:23-32. This gospel reading is in two parts. When Jesus is asked about his authority before answering he asks the chief priests where John's baptism came from which they cannot answer because they were too worldly and afraid of what the people would think. Then he hits back at them with another question about the two sons the one who said he would do something and didn't and the other who said we wouldn't but did so who did what the father asked, and then condemned them for not listening to John or himself while the tax collectors and prostitutes did.

If authority and status is only worldly it is empty for all the show and supposed importance people with it have, knowing the right people and going to the right meetings may get you promotions but what does it all mean because to climb the ladder often means walking on other people. The people who count in God's eyes are the ones who make mistakes but are humble enough to know their faults and admit them and realise they have to trust in God, the people who actually do what God has asked and cared for others. Jesus knew the leaders of his day would not listen because they believed in themselves rather than God, so his message was to the people who flocked to hear him in their thousands, they recognised his authority without having to ask. True authority comes from God and you will recognise it when you see it, we all know who is genuine and if God has spoken to you in these difficult times then you are the ones with authority, you are the ones chosen by God.

Kingsley

Mon 28 Sept

Subject: Week 27

Dear Friends

What I particularly liked about Bishop Joanna coming to Cyffig yesterday was the very Celtic feel of the whole thing. The Bishop was on her way to St David's Cathedral for an Ordination and stopped off at a small out of the way church with a small congregation to Confirm one person, there was no great show, no fuss, and it was her joy to do this, she was not too important. It was a simple, casual service which meant so very much to those who were there. It seems one of the positive by-products of this partial lockdown is the smaller, more intimate gatherings which are far more meaningful than packing the church. Even the fact that the Bishop is a woman was very Celtic because the Celtic Church did have women Bishops.

Is this the future of the church? Simpler, more local, less staid and stuffy. We will see.

Kingsley

Tues 29 Sept

Dear Friends

29th September, Michael and All Angels, so I think a few words about angels would be applicable today.

- First sphere: 1. Seraphim, 2. Cherubim, 3. Thrones;
- Second sphere: 4. Dominations (also translated as Lordships), 5. Virtues (also trans. as Powers), 6. Powers (also trans. as Authorities);
- Third sphere: 7. Principalities, 8. Archangels, 9. **Angels.**

The first sphere are the angels whose job it is to worship God constantly. The second oversee the universe and all matter, protect it against evil, they guide the planets and the very atoms of nature. The third guide and protect us, they are the messengers. The Principalities oversee nations, Archangels humanity as a whole, Angels deal with us directly on a personal level.

They cannot go against God's plan or our free will but they have powers we cannot begin to understand. It is this ninth rank that the guardian angels come in. I have mentioned that there is an angel in St Mary's but that our idea of being in a place is different to the reality of the angel who is actually in the spiritual realm but has a presence there, the same as guardian angels although they are with us they are also constantly in the presence of God. And this is where it gets complicated, we are in the presence of God too but don't always realise it. There is so much more going on than we can ever know, we are never alone. Our eyes are closed to the wonders that surround us and even when we go through sadness and pain and loss we are not abandoned.

Kingsley

Wed 30 Sept

Dear Friends

Do you know why we drive on the left? It goes back to the days when people rode horses, they would pass each other on the left so they could shake hands with their right hand. So how did people on the continent greet each other on horseback? So many of the things we take for granted have a reason way back in history. So many of the things we do in church have strange histories and very often nothing to do with religion or the Bible. When a couple come from church having been married the groom walks on the right so he can protect his bride with his sword arm (assuming he is not left handed). The clerical collar has no religious significance at all, it goes back to a twelfth Century hunting collar.

This isn't to say that we should simply discard tradition, after all tradition is familiar and comforting especially in an ever changing world. I will admit I am not a great fan of change and very often changes are made for no good reason. We need to think carefully before we change anything, is it actually better? The world has changed out of necessity and will continue to do so for a while yet. It is not better now but I trust that the ultimate change will be better. A new church is emerging with many of the large showy events being replaced by smaller more intimate ones, we are getting back to a more local church which relies on the people who are the backbone of the church anyway. As more churches open again in this group it is because the people are quite capable of doing so. You are the church and you are the future.

Kingsley

Thu 1 Oct

Dear Friends

It isn't all gloom. Many places are in lockdown and the PM is threatening a complete lockdown but the Imperial College of London says the present measures are working and the Bank of England chief says the economy is bouncing back.

Even in areas where there is lockdown the places of worship are still open. The people waiting to go into the paper shop this morning were cheerful and upbeat.

The sun is shining and the early mist that settled in the valley is clearing. The world still rolls its way around the sun and the seasons still follow each other. Harvest services are still taking place, Lampeter Velfrey had theirs outside, St Mary's are celebrating this coming Sunday and Cyffig and Clydai the Sunday after even if they are smaller events, and nothing is going to dampen our enthusiasm, we are not giving in to fear and doom and gloom. Harvest festival is as old as farming and is ingrained into the fibre of our being, to thank God for all that he has done for us and to look forward with hope to the future.

Kingsley

Fri 2 Oct

Dear Friends

I suppose many of you have noticed by now that I am a little bit nutty and my feet are not firmly on the ground. Having said that I can be very organised when I need to be or I wouldn't have got the position I have. I am also very fascinated by folklore, myth and legend. There has to be some truth at the heart of every tale and every saying somewhere, and there is possibly something we can learn from it.

What we can see in this world is not all that there is, human beings have always believed there was something more, something beyond, and they have always tried to make sense of it. I was talking about angels a few days ago, it is worth noting that when Lucifer was cast out of heaven and became Satan he took a third of the angels with him who are the demons, therefore there are two thirds who are still angels. Not only are there twice as many angels as demons but there is no evil opposite of God. I don't know where the balance of good and evil comes from because it is not an equal balance, there is far more good in this world than evil, there are far more good people than bad, there is more hope than despair, more love than hate. If there is a battle then evil is already on the losing side. No matter how dark the days are, no matter how much fear, there is so much more that is better to come. If times are hard for you now, hang in there, tomorrow is bright.

Kingsley

Sat 3 Oct

Dear Friends

I am grateful to Roslyn who sends me her Sunday resources all the way from Montreal because this time she talks about St Francis of Assisi, in the Church in Wales lectionary because his feast day is on Sunday he is completely overlooked and as he is one of my favourite saints I would have been very sad to miss him out. So I would like to make it up to him today.

St Francis had a very privileged background but when he discovered a small ruined church was told to rebuild the church by Jesus, but this was not just the ruin rather the church as a whole that had lost its way. He gave up everything to live a simple life, he became very close to nature in all its aspects and is patron saint of animals and the environment. In his love for the whole of creation he saw it as much more than a lifeless thing, he saw God in everything. It is interesting that he saw God work through Brother Sun, Sister Moon, Brother Wind, Sister Water, etc.

It seems that every once in a while God likes to remind the church of a simpler faith because it has a habit of getting caught up in pomp and ceremony and its own importance. And this is where we are again now, although this time it is not through a vision to one person but a wake-up call to all who are willing to listen and have eyes to see. Now is the time for us all to rebuild the church.

Kingsley

Sun 4 Oct

Subject: Trinity 17

Dear Friends

Matthew 21: 33-46. The parable of the tenants of the vineyard who beat or killed the owners' representatives when they came to collect the fruit, so he sent his son and the tenants killed the son so they could inherit the vineyard. The chief priests and Pharisees knew he was talking about them because God often referred to the people of Israel as his vineyard throughout the Old Testament. The implication here is that the Jewish authorities knew perfectly well that Jesus was God's son and that by killing him they could do without God. History is full of arrogant people who thought they were so powerful they could take over the world and live for ever, yet all the great empires of the past have gone.

Even in smaller ways so many people strive for power over others and for what? Power is fleeting as is status and influence, our true treasure is in heaven and it is our standing with God that is important. It is only by obeying his command to love that we gain eternal life and in heaven no one is greater than anyone else. Do not seek to puff yourself up and put others down, enjoy life for what God has given you, each of us has an important part to play and we all need each other.

Kingsley

Mon 5 Oct

Subject: Week 28

Dear Friends

Along with a harvest service in St Mary's, with thanks to all who brought produce, three more churches in the LMA had their first service yesterday, with thanks to the wardens. Whatever else the church is re-emerging as a presence in our communities and is a beacon of hope and as long as we are sensible it will continue to be so.

This doesn't mean I am going to stop writing these emails or even begin to wind down, I am afraid now

I have started getting me to stop is going to be very difficult. We are still going through difficult times and the winter is ahead, but we have to get through winter to arrive at spring.

The early settlers here, possibly the Mesolithic hunter gatherers, would have to store as much food as they could at this time of year to see them through the winter, for them the winters were harder because they had just come out of the last ice age. They survived, they settled, they grew, they developed, they became farmers and they expanded and I often wonder how many of the local people could trace their ancestry right back to them. We too will get through the winter, we always do, and spring will come again. While the earth remains, seedtime and harvest, cold and heat, summer and winter, day and night, shall not cease. (Gen 8.22)

Kingsley

Tue 6 Oct

Dear Friends

One of the things the Archdeacon always puts in his bulletins is the insistence that clergy should take a holiday. Obviously because everyone is different the idea of holiday is going to be different for everyone. I would absolutely hate to lie on the beach in the sun, I could not bear just to lounge around I have one of those restless minds that has to be stimulated all the time. Fortunately Jo-an and I like the same sort of holiday, to go away somewhere remote away from everything but a place that has plenty to explore. We have been to so many of the Scottish Islands like Shetland, Orkney, the Outer Hebrides, Skye etc. Holiday is a break from the normal, a change. In many ways I don't feel I need a holiday this year because since March it has been a break from the normal and I have found plenty to stimulate my restless mind.

Our journey through this pandemic has been just that, a journey, and it is ongoing. Almost an adventure. There are dangers along the way, there is sadness and loss, there is uncertainty, but it is all a new experience for everyone, and although we don't know where we are going because there is no map we know we will get there sometime. There is promise ahead and possibly even treasure, certainly much to celebrate in time and joy to be had. Thank you for coming with me.

Kingsley

Wed 7 Oct

Dear Friends

Ps 98.9 Let the rivers clap their hands, let the mountains sing together for joy. Is 55.13b the mountains and hills will burst into song before you, and all the trees of the field will clap their hands. Luke 19.40 "I tell you," he replied, "if they keep quiet, the stones will cry out."

The whole of nature doesn't just reflect the glory of God, nature itself glories in God and not in a passive way. St Francis of Assisi knew this and so did the Celtic church. When we live in harmony with nature we are in closer harmony with God, The Maker Of All Things. When we see the whole of reality as one then there is no division between physical and spiritual, we will see the spiritual flow through everything because everything is of God, then we will understand miracles as part of the natural world around us and they will not be a matter of faith or belief but part of life.

We have seen what happens when humans tamper with nature as if it is a commodity to be used. It is time we listened to nature and respected it.

Kingsley

Thu 8 Oct

Dear Friends

With so many different views on the best way to deal with this pandemic no wonder we are all confused. When the rules keep changing it is difficult to keep up. For all the expert advice it seems as if everyone is stumbling about in the dark. Hindsight would be useful about now, unfortunately it doesn't work like that but in the future people will have enough to say about what should have been done. Everyone is so wise after the event, to live through an event like this is a day at a time.

We are not going to lose hope though, we will get through this together, and even as we live in these times there are plenty of things to rejoice about. The future may be uncertain but there is still a future ahead of us, the world isn't about to end. And for those who would like the world to end remember that Jesus prayed in the garden that we might have the full measure of joy within us even in this world. God is the only constant in this world and we reach out to him for peace and joy and hope. We all have a part to play in encouraging and supporting each other, so let us do just that.

Kingsley

Fri 9 Oct

Dear Friends

There are times and situations where we feel powerless, where we seem to have no choice. But this is not really so. We always have a choice, we can choose how we deal with situations we are in. Our present lives seem to be driven by the pandemic and the rules the government give keep changing. But there is no point moaning about it, that won't change anything and it only makes us more miserable and drag others down with us. Rather look for the things that we can do, the choices we can make.

We can still go to the shops and talk to people while we queue, we can still phone our family and friends, we can still send emails and the more computer literate can Skype or Zoom or whatever. We can still meet in church (even if we can't sing) and we can have some sort of fellowship (2m). We can laugh and smile we can love, we can hope and dream. No one can take away who we are and who God designed us to be. We can live our lives.

Live life today

Kingsley

Sat 10 Oct

Subject: Hello from your friendly LMA Dean

Dear Friends

Apart from today I dropped LMA from the subject line because these emails are hardly just the LMA any more. You will also notice that they have been called Reflections for some time and that needs a little explanation.

I am sorry for being secretive, evasive or dismissive about a certain issue that so many of you have mentioned, but there have been plans to publish a book for some time now and I didn't want to mention it until the book was actually available. It will also be available in Waterstones in Carmarthen although they couldn't arrange a book signing under the present circumstances. I didn't know what to call the book but Jo-an, who has been encouraging and supporting me throughout, suggested Reflections, the emails in the book had to stop just after the open air service in Whitland because I had to stop somewhere when submitting it to the publisher, and it has taken all this time to get it to the press. It is interesting in that it is a reminder of how things were from the beginning of the lockdown.

Meanwhile, on with volume 2. The journey continues and there are possibly hard times to come, some of the stories you hear of people unable to visit loved ones in hospital or care homes are heart-breaking, the road has been very rough. We must continue to draw on our own strength and be willing to draw on the strength of others. We know God is with us but it is very hard to realise he is there at times and although Jesus was human we need the physical presence of other human beings. Being willing to open up to others, to admit weakness is a risky business because there are those who would capitalise on it, but there are so many good people in the world who will genuinely be there for you. Accept help when it is offered and watch for need in those around you and together we will get through the winter and it will be spring again.

Kingsley

Sun 11 Oct

Subject: Trinity 18

Dear Friends

Philippians 4.1-9. After asking a few people to actually get on with each other Paul begins 'Rejoice in the Lord always ...' and continues in the most positive way in any of his letters, well worth a read, telling his readers to look for and think of all the positive things. This is a reading we can try and take to heart today.

Don't look for fault in each other, don't spoil for an argument but look for good. Think about all the positive things in your life at the moment and give yourself hope. Do the kind and thoughtful things for others. Smile (under your mask). Complement one another. In doing this we can brighten the day not only for others but for ourselves as well. Expect this to be a good day.

Kingsley

Mon 12 Oct

Subject: Week 29

Dear Friends

It was good to be invited to the re-opening of St Clydai yesterday evening which was also their harvest festival, another step forward, and if anyone doesn't know the church it is worth going to have a look as it is like a small cathedral. With all the backward steps taking place at the moment it is good to report any forward steps.

There is a light drizzle this morning, the leaves of the trees are turning to their vibrant autumn colours, the ground it littered with acorns, everywhere nature is preparing for winter. Whatever we feel about winter it is part of our rhythm in this part of the world and the changing seasons add colour and variety to our lives, I for one wouldn't live anywhere else. And so is life, life is ups and downs, the hard times build strength and help us to appreciate the good times. We have to go through so many different experiences or life is just an existence. When we go through difficulties, loss and sadness perhaps we would wish these times didn't happen but everything adds to who we are and when we come through them we feel more alive. These messages I have deliberately kept positive, not because I have not known sadness, pain and loss but because we all need encouragement and hope at this time and because I am a raving optimist. Today is full of possibilities, enjoy today.

Kingsley

Tue 13 Oct

Dear Friends

I had a funeral yesterday, I didn't know the woman nor the family, they moved into the area some years ago, and yet I found it as sad as if I had known them. If only everyone viewed every death whether near of far, known or unknown as a sad happening, especially now with the number of COVID-19 deaths seen as a statistic. If only everyone was aware of everyone else's worries and concerns. Yet I have seen the concern people have shown for neighbours during this time, the good that previous strangers have done. There is a lot of quiet, genuine goodness in humanity which is why the selfish and thoughtless stand out. Now is the time to reach out and embrace those around us even if we can't physically, we cannot set ourselves apart or put ourselves on pedestals because we are all going through this. The good that is done in the community is not paraded around or boasted about, it is done simply without fuss.

Another thing that makes me sad is that we cannot sing. During the World Wars songs were written and sung to inspire and encourage. There don't seem to have been any rousing songs written, and nothing we could sing together even if we were allowed. We desperately need to sing together to raise our spirits. My main prayer at the moment (other than an end to the virus) is that singing will be pronounced safe. Still, we can sing in our minds and our hearts, there is always music going on in my head. And there are more things that bring me joy than bring me sadness, I still rejoice and I am still welling up with hope.

Rejoice in the good things today.

Kingsley

Wed 14 Oct

Dear Friends

Back in March we didn't know how long this was going to last and in the summer as restrictions were slowly lifted we dared to hope we were over the worst even though we were being warned of a second wave and a hard winter. Now we are in the second wave and winter is looming. But now is not the time to lose hope and give in to fear and depression. We were in the eye of the storm and we made the most of it, now we are coming back into the storm and although things look dark keep your eyes open for the star that breaks through the cloud.

Even areas with a hard lockdown places of worship remain open, so let us hope that continues after all the hard work people have put in to opening their churches again, we were denied Easter let us hope we will not be denied Christmas.

All of us in our lives have weathered storms before, this present storm we are not expected to weather alone but we do so together. As in the two World Wars this is a time when we realise we need each other. There is a strength and resilience in communities and no storm lasts for ever. Batten down the hatches, forge ahead, and we will get to the calm waters and the safe haven.

Kingsley

Thu 15 Oct

Dear Friends

Yesterday I had my 5 free copies of the book and started to read it. I don't think it hit me until then just how these simple messages have taken off. I had hoped to go to St Non's for a few days recently (I could have still written these on my iPad from there) only with the second wave the Nuns had to cancel all retreats, I would have liked to sit on the cliff top again and recall the discussion (mostly one sided) I had with God just before my Ordination, the discussion that ended with me saying I could not do this without him and his only ever answer of 'Good'. Because I find myself in that same place now, these emails I could not do without him. But

I suppose what he is saying is that I do not need to go to St Non's for he is still with me.

On Palm Sunday I objected to the glib answer to where is God in all this and admitted I do not know (read the book!). I suppose he is with us but it still doesn't answer the question fully. My messages are not the answer simply the struggle. But this I do know, if we reach out to him he is there even if he doesn't answer our questions, and in the end he himself will wipe the tears from our eyes, I only hope he has some big hankies because we all have a lot of tears. And this also I know, we will get through this, he has made nature strong enough to fight back at whatever humanity does and nature will make us more resilient to the virus.

Hold on

Kingsley

Fri 16 Oct

Dear Friends

The Welsh Government are talking about a circuit breaker for Wales with details to follow. I expect this is filling a lot of people with dread. We can only take this one day at a time. As I said recently we have all had to face difficult patches in our lives it is just that this time we face it together.

One day we will be able to look back at this, and it is not that far in the future, and time will heal some of the anguish and fear. We will be able to sing again and we will be able to cwtch again. We will have our stories to tell to those who come after, the memory of this time will live long into the future but it will lose its sting. For the moment though don't give in to fear, look for joy along the way, smile and laugh. Believe in magic. Trust yourselves and each other, we are all better and stronger than we think. Never lose hope.

Kingsley

Sat 17 Oct

Dear Friends

Moving from The Vicarage into Y Ficerdy last year was useful in that I had to throw a lot of stuff away. And as anyone who has moved you still end up with a lot of stuff in boxes for a long time after. So I am still going through things and getting rid of things. Unfortunately I am a dreadful hoarder and everything seems to have a memory attached to it and there are things I really do not need but still can't get rid of.

Computers these days have a large amount of memory but even that is not finite and when I start looking for old files I find I have to wade through a lot of files I do not need and some time I will have to start deleting things.

But the human brain does seem to be limitless, it stores all the memories, all the things we have seen or done or read or heard or learned and we cannot clear those things out. You never hear of anyone whose brain is so full it cannot take in anything more. It is so sad when a wasting disease starts taking these memories away and you can't pick and choose which ones.

For those who understand such things you can back up your computer, tablet or smartphone on the cloud but your memories? Your memories are stored too, our spiritual selves are not limited to our physical bodies and it is comforting to know that we will get all our memories back. Our memories are a great part of who we are, they are a well of treasures and experiences good and bad, and each day we make more memories, make your experiences good ones today.

Kingsley

Sun 18 Oct

Subject: Luke, Evangelist

Dear Friends

Luke is an interesting character for several reasons. He was not Jewish for a start, he was a Greek doctor and travelled with Paul on some of his journeys first meeting up with him at Troas and we only know this because as author of Acts in relating Paul's journey he changes from they to we. His gospel has several things that the others don't so it is obvious that although he wasn't a witness he talked to many who were including Mary, Jesus' mother. And we know he was with Paul at the end of his ministry while others had left him. Luke was a steady person who was always there and didn't push himself forward.

Not everyone needs to make a big thing of what they have done, just to be there for others and quietly get on with things. I have found this everywhere, it is not the people who make a show of their good deeds who are the best people, it is the people who do so much for others without fanfare who really make a difference. I may have written a book but it is all of you who are the salt and light in the world.

Kingsley

Mon 19 Oct

Subject: Week 30

Dear Friends

I have just had a delivery of 30 books, stop me and buy one.

Later today the First Minister will be announcing whether we will be in lockdown from Friday and what will be affected. I found yesterday's service quite sad because if the churches are closed again, even if only for a few weeks, it means all we have accomplished has stopped, I hope that when the lockdown is relaxed the risk assessments forms we have already done will still be valid. But we do not know yet what will happen so I am not going to expect the worst.

We got through the first lockdown I am sure we can manage this, whatever it is.

When we were first required to wear face masks I found it quite fiddly, now I can slip it on quite easily. Unfortunately it makes my ears stick out, one person said it makes me look like a pixie. I have got a selection of different ones, most of you have seen the smiley face, and apart from the East Landsker one that I was kindly given I am not going to wear a religious one because I am not religious and I am certainly not holy. If there is one thing that annoys me it is holy people! We are all human beings with our faults, we are all good and bad, not one of us is perfect yet with God's help we can all be better than we are. Life is a journey not a destination, those who think they have arrived only fool themselves. Do not put yourself down and never let anyone else put you down either.

Hold your head up today.

Kingsley

Part 4
Second Lockdown

Tue 20 Oct

Dear Friends

So now we know, there is a temporary lockdown from Friday and the Churches will be closed along with a lot of other things. They are calling this a circuit breaker but I don't understand the term in this context, why stick fancy words on things when everyone knows what a lockdown is now.

I did say recently that we got through the last lockdown so we will get through this too. We have learned to cope with the strange world we live in now where the rules change all the time, this time we know what to do because we have the support of our communities and our friends, we can face anything. This is not as severe anyway, it is more of a precaution in a way with winter coming up. So we grit our teeth, forge ahead and see this through. We continue to look for the good things each day and grasp the joys as they come and we look forward with eager hope for there are even better days to come.

I believe in you.

Kingsley

Wed 21 Oct

Dear Friends

I like mystery, I like the fact that we cannot know everything about anything, even if we are an expert in a particular area we will still not know it all even about our own subject. I like the fact that there is always so much more to learn. The picture on the cover of the book is of the moon and her reflection in water. The moon is mysterious enough and the reflection, although it is of the moon, is broken into pieces on the ripples of the water, and I was thinking that this is how we see God.

God is unknowable anyway and our image of him is in pieces and not one of us has all the pieces, we can only know God truly in this life through the experiences everyone has of him. 1 Cor 13.12 Now we see but a poor reflection as in a mirror; ... In those days they didn't have mirrors as we know them only highly polished metal surfaces which only gave a poor reflection. If we hold too tightly to a set of beliefs we have already decided then certain experiences in life can blow this apart. God himself doesn't change but we have to accept he is greater than our understanding of him. As I listen to other people's experiences I learn more about God, listen to others today and get from them more of the pieces.

Kingsley

Thu 22 Oct

Dear Friends

It is interesting that the reaction of people to this second lockdown are so mixed. On the one hand the virus is still around, though far less dangerous because medicines have improved, and we still need to be cautious, on the other hand people are getting weary. In either case I am still here if you need me which is where I started in March and will continue to give hope, this time I have far more emails that I send to quite apart from those who send this message to others.

After all the hard work people put in to opening their churches again it is a little disappointing that they are all closed again, but they are prepared and can open again once this is over and there is an excellent chance we will be able to celebrate Christmas in them.

Last night Deanna treated Jo-an, myself and the three youngest boys to supper in Carmarthen. We had such fun, the boys are so comical and so caring of each other, this was an absolute joy. And this is the secret to getting through hard times, family. Also friends, neighbours and the community. I bet Jesus had a lot of fun too which we tend to forget. Laugh, enjoy life, look forward with hope, dream, have fun today.

Kingsley

Fri 23 Oct

Dear Friends

It seems strange that I am not preparing for Sunday again, normally (well normally for the present) I would be changing the psalm in the power point service and emailing or telephoning someone to ask them to read. I am adrift again, not knowing what day of the week it is.

You all know me well enough by now to know that I do not know the meaning of despair, so I will use this temporary pause as a time to slow down and reflect. It may be raining and the distant hills grey and insubstantial but it is still a new day and we can still look for something good. Today is the last day before lockdown but we have been here before and we know what to do, make the most of the time ahead and we will get on with things again very soon. Life will go on, we can get out even if it means coats, we can still talk as we queue outside shops even if we don't know who we are talking to with masks and hoods. Alexa tells me Christmas is in 63 days and Christmas is the day God showed he wanted to experience what we experience and became one of us, we do not live in an unfeeling universe.

Kingsley

Sat 24 Oct

Dear Friends

In Wales we are in lockdown again and although we were warned we dared to believe we were over the worst. We are over the worst and this is only a temporary measure but we feel this is dragging on. If only we could fast forward a year, look back at this and enjoy being free again. "There'll be bluebirds over the white cliffs of Dover tomorrow, just you wait and see."

Meanwhile, we continue to support each other, share the love and hope, smile beneath our masks, talk at a distance. Keep calm and carry on. Yesterday as I tapped away it was wet and miserable and not long after the day opened up and was gloriously sunny, bad weather passes. Bad times pass and there is always more joy and happiness. We need to be understanding of others who do find these times hard and share our well of hope with them.

Kingsley

Sun 25 Oct

Subject: Bible Sunday

Dear Friends

Matthew 24:30-35. The end of the world is nigh! Except it isn't. For all the so called prophets of doom who examine the Bible and fit the things that have happened or are happening in the world around what they see as predictions the end still hasn't happened. Only when we see Jesus return in power will we know for sure. I do find this a strange reading to have on Bible Sunday. I like the new testament reading Col 3:12-17 because it tells us how we should live now, it talks of compassion, kindness, humility, gentleness, patience, forgiveness and love. If only people wouldn't have their preconceived ideas and make the Bible fit round them and concentrate on living the way God asks there would be fewer rifts, disagreements, wars, etc.

I will miss Church today, it is seen as non-essential, but what about spiritual wellbeing, mental health, companionship. There has been such joy when people have been able to gather together for worship and I am sure we in Wales all feel the loss today. But we can still be together in a spiritual sense, think of all the unknown number who read this with you today and realise you are part of something even if not physically together. God can draw us together in love and hope.

Peace

Kingsley

Mon 26 Oct

Subject: Week 31

Dear Friends

Every day for 31 weeks I have sat here and looked out over the valley, I watched the new spring leaves, the wild flowers, the wind and the rain and the sunshine, the blackberries and apples, the changing colours of the leaves and now their falling. I have never experienced a year so long nor been able to stand back and watch in so much detail. With so much sadness in the world we are surrounded by the glories of nature, it is a wonderful world if only we looked after it and ourselves better.

I have a great respect for nature, it is a living thing and it is an outpouring of God's creativity. There are many things human beings need, space, time, wonder, companionship. We do not need objects except the basics, we do not need power, we do not need to fill our lives with stuff that drag us down. Take time to look after yourself today.

Kingsley

Tue 27 Oct

Dear Friends

We have all learned so much through this pandemic, our lives have changed several times, we have found we need each other so much more. We have had to find a resilience deep within ourselves, and as this drags on into the winter we need to dig deeper again. But we need to remember there will be an end, the virus may not go away but it will be just one among many like the flu, we will deal with it as we deal with everything. We will pick up the pieces, put fear behind us and get on with living.

For all the restrictions that are in place at the moment we can still dream and hope and love. We may not be able to sing but there is still music, I find I sing a lot in the car because I do not want to find that when we can sing in Church my voice has gone. There is art and poetry and books, there is beauty all around us, don't look down at the ground but raise your eyes and look around even when it is raining.

See wonders today.

Kingsley

Wed 28 Oct

Dear Friends

Everyone I speak to says this lockdown feels different, there is a weariness with people, it is as if everyone was becoming hopeful and their hopes are dashed. Last time the rules were simple, now they are so complicated. Last time it was spring and the weather was glorious and now we face the winter.

Ps 23:4 Even though I walk through the valley of the shadow of death, I will fear no evil, for you are with me; your rod and your staff, they comfort me.

There is also the hope of a vaccine getting closer, and I am here at the end of an email if you need me. Do not lose heart, do not give in to depression, do not fear. Reach out to one another, we will get through this together.

Every blessing

Kingsley

Thu 29 Oct

Dear Friends

Technology has been very useful at this time but it is not perfect and we shouldn't always rely on it. I have had to restart my computer this morning because it wasn't working properly, the times I have gone to pay in a shop and the person behind the till has complained at the slowness of the system or the system is down. Did you know that when sorting out a computer problem is called debugging it is because an early fault with an early computer an insect (bug for the Americans) had got into it. For all the wonders of technology it still inhabits the real world.

Although I am basically a shy person and can cope on my own I do enjoy company, I like people. Not everyone I have to admit despite the Bible telling me I should. At the moment I am having to content myself with talking to people queueing up for shops and chatting to shopkeepers. It must be really hard for people who can't get out, I feel for them. Next year there will be such joy when people can mix again, shake hands, hug, cwtch. All the things you can't do over the internet, you can't do on Facebook, you can't do on zoom. Do not become distant and afraid during this time, there is still joy even now.

Kingsley

Fri 30 Oct

Dear Friends

I have often likened what we are going through as a journey or a pilgrimage, and I am thankful to those of you who have taken the trouble to respond with stories of you own with the things you have been doing. The road ahead is still a long one and we can still use this opportunity to learn. Every experience we go through in life adds to what we know, and very often the journey is learning as much about ourselves as anything else. In fact a pilgrimage is always more of an inward journey even when the pilgrims physically travel, but this pilgrimage more so because we are not going to an actual destination and there is no map.

Because I have been doing most of the 'talking' I expect you have all learned a lot about me that you didn't already know. For instance I am slightly dyslectic, something readers of the book won't know because the spellings are put right in that, which probably explains my sometimes disorganised thinking. And during this second lockdown I have had to reflect a lot more again and who knows I may yet reveal more of my inner thoughts, how my feet are not firmly on the ground and I am always a bit of a dreamer and this is why I can be so positive all the time. I hope none of you are psychologists! But the hope I have is not because of my rose coloured spectacles but because of experience, things are never as bad as we think they are going to be. We have all got through hard times before, we become stronger and we appreciate all the things that are good. No matter what, today is a good day.

Kingsley

Sat 31 Oct

Dear Friends

Samhain (pronounced saun) is an old Celtic festival, possibly even earlier, that starts this evening and ends tomorrow evening. It is a time when this world and the otherworld are closer so families would gather together and remember deceased members of the family and when I say remember in this context celebrate a meal together with them. Then comes the Christian Church and in its typical fashion overlay this festival with another, All Saints and rather than celebrate with deceased family they celebrate with the important people of the past. On top of this comes dressing up as ghosts and ghouls and witches etc. and the American habit of trick or treat, nothing to do with it at all. So I am glad that in Wales at least this has been curtailed.

Where does this leave us then? Everyone has lost loved ones, but they are not gone and rather than think of evil spirits this evening raise a glass to absent friends. If the veil between us and the otherworld is thinner then it brings us closer to the heavenly realm with rank upon rank of angels who are there to protect us and not scare us. And perhaps we can see God clearer too. Throw away thoughts of darkness and seek the light.

Happy All Hallows Eve

Kingsley

Sun 1 Nov

Subject: All Saints

Dear Friends

Matthew 5. 1-12. This is the beginning of the sermon on the mount, the part when Jesus says all those 'Blessed are ..' statements. The whole sermon runs for three chapters and the impression I have always had was this was delivered to ordinary people and the promises were to everyone. Jesus never ranked people according to goodness but treated everyone the same, the reward of eternal life was always a free gift and not something to be earned. So I have never understood why the church has had All Saints today and All Souls tomorrow as if there is going to be a two tier system in heaven. The only hierarchy is God and even he came to this world to serve. We are so hung up on status and position and the church is no exception and this is not God's way.

You are loved by God and special to him, you are neither superior nor inferior to anyone else. Don't let anyone look down on you nor should you look down on anyone else.

All Saints Day was set up because there were not enough days in the year to give all the people the Church deemed saints to give them all a day. But as we are all equal in God's eyes then we can celebrate our own saints day on our birthday, so if it someone's birthday today then happy saints day to you.

Every blessing

Kingsley

Mon 2 Nov

Subject: Week 32

Dear Friends

In Wales we are half way through the lockdown but England are facing a month's long lockdown and there is the possibility of another lockdown here. And I am sure the other countries this goes to are facing problems too. So much of our lives have been put on hold yet few people can really afford to do so. There will be an end but can we see the light at the end of the tunnel yet, it is going on and on. And there will be long term health and financial issues to deal with.

But life does go on, there are joys to be had, there are things to celebrate. We are still here for one another, to do the practical things, to encourage and to give hope. We have all faced difficulties before, now we face them together and draw strength from one another. We have all found ways to cope and we will continue to do so. One day we will look back on this and be proud of what we have done.

Be strong

Kingsley

Tue 3 Nov

Dear Friends

After writing these emails I go down to Whitland for the paper, walking when I can, so I don't know today's news yet. But yesterday's paper was all doom and gloom. Where are the rallying calls, where are the stirring speeches of hope? If there have been some either from the state or the church then I have missed them, if someone can point out some that I have missed let me know.

Stirring speech or not we are not going to give in, we will not be beaten down by fear. We will continue to hope and dream and love and laugh. We will get through our present difficulties with determination and win this battle too. I will continue to wave my little flag and wherever you are wave yours as well, let us be bright beacons in this dark world, a centre for hope in our communities. We are the church whether the buildings are open or closed, we are ambassadors of heaven.

Keep calm and carry on

Kingsley

Wed 4 Nov

Dear Friends

What a strange world we live in at the moment. Not only are all sorts of places taped up like a crime scene, even our churches, but everyone is going about with masks like bank robbers. During a war we know who the enemy is, we can see maps where land is gained and lost, we know when it is over because a treaty is signed and we can celebrate. In this war the enemy is unseen, statistics are well known to be manipulated to prove whatever you want, and the virus will always be there but it will be just one among many that we will deal with and life will return to some sort of normal so gradually that we won't know when to celebrate.

When we no longer wear masks, when we can mix with whomever we want, when we can cwtch, when we can sing, especially when the larger lady does. When the song in our hearts can burst forth from our lips, then the celebration will not just be a one off party but the rest of our lives appreciating all that we have. In the meantime keep the song in your heart alive, the smile on your lips under the mask, appreciate the things we do have even now. Continue to give thanks and drive the darkness away.

I wish you joy today

Kingsley

Thu 5 Nov

Dear Friends

Remember, remember the fifth of November, gunpowder treason and plot. I never met Guy Fawkes and his attempt to blow up the houses of Parliament was before my time, so how can I remember? My memories of the fifth of November as a child were standing in our back garden, my father taking fireworks from the box one by one, reading what it was called with a torch, taking it down the garden and setting it off, Catherine wheels never working, waving sparklers in our gloved hands and drinking soup from a mug. Surely the event, important though it was at the time, has no relevance to us today.

Remembrance day on the other hand is not only about an event still in living memory but it is a reminder of sacrifice and why we should never go to war again, it will always be relevant.

I wonder how our present troubles will be remembered and what lessons can be learned. Will we learn not to tamper with nature? Will there be a day to remember those who died, and what about those who suffered, those who lost their livelihoods, etc.?

But for us now it is too soon to think about that because we are living through it. Today is another day we have been given and must be enjoyed to the full.

Kingsley

Fri 6 Nov

Dear Friends

On a pilgrimage it isn't supposed to be one long hard slog, there are places along the way where you can be refreshed and you can relax a little. I have mentioned before that people on a pilgrimage to St David's Cathedral would have camped out over night at the chapel of ease where St Mary's is now and local people and hostellers (the equivalent of Mike Station House!) would have supplied them with sustenance. Ours is a pilgrimage even though some of you have been with us from the beginning while others have joined along the way (at least you can read the book if you missed the earlier emails). I know from your replies that at times it has been a hard slog and at other times there has been fun and I have enjoyed your stories too.

On a physical pilgrimage those who complete it arrive at their destination (such as St David's) there would be a service led by the Dean or the Bishop and there would be a celebration. How will we mark the end of our pilgrimage? When will we know we have arrived? What would be wonderful if those of us who could get to St David's would meet there and perhaps the Bishop could give an address.

In the meantime, take whatever opportunities you can to rest and enjoy yourself.

Every Blessing

Kingsley

Sat 7 Nov

Dear Friends

Time is still an enigma to me. This year continues to seemingly go on for ever. Time always drags when you are waiting and we are waiting now. We are waiting for an end but of what? We know the virus will always be with us but we will have a vaccine and the virus will melt into the background. We are waiting for and end of lockdown but for those in England it has just started and for us in Wales we don't know when another will be imposed. We are waiting to have freedom to meet up with people again but we don't know when that will be. So we wait for and end that we will not be able to define even when it comes. And this waiting is putting a strain on so many people

I must be odd, I am probably rather annoying too, because I seem to have a well of joy within me that will not stop and I have such a hope that cannot be dampened. It is not that the cares and concerns of others don't touch me, I feel them deeply, I do find it hard not to cry at funerals I take, I get upset when I see people suffer. But there is still this well of joy and I don't know where it comes from, there is always a song in my heart.

I am waiting too, but I am getting on with living. Each day is unique and should be enjoyed for what it brings.

Kingsley

Sun 8 Nov

Subject: Remembrance

Dear Friends

A hundred years ago the Unknown Warrior was buried at Westminster Abbey to lie with kings to represent all the soldiers who died during World War I. Today at cenotaphs and war memorials all over the country the names of the soldiers from each local community will be read out and remembered. Every life is important. Every death affects friends and families. Such is the sadness of this world, that people we love die and one day we must leave the people we love too.

Do not think God doesn't understand, that God doesn't feel, even though he knows that after death we come to him. When Lazarus died Jesus went out of his way to comfort his sisters and even though he knew he would raise him from the dead he was moved to tears and we have the shortest verse in the whole Bible, 'Jesus wept', and this verse in its simplicity says so much. As we struggle with the questions on why God allows certain things hold on to this verse. I said in one of my first emails that I do not know the answer, I still don't. But this verse is the closest we are going to get.

So live, appreciate each day, appreciate all your friends and family and live.

Kingsley

Mon 9 Nov

Subject: Week 33

Dear Friends

I don't know about everywhere else but in Whitland the weather was dry yesterday and we were able to hold a Remembrance Day service outside the Memorial Hall, we were limited to numbers and the cars passing didn't help so I found it a particularly sad occasion. Still, we marked the day and we remembered those from the community who gave their lives.

Today, we in Wales come out of lockdown but there are certain restrictions now that didn't apply before. However for services of worship in Church we are not restricted to the 15 people rule but the safe capacity that we already had, this is a relief as I didn't want to have to turn anyone away.

We still cannot sing.

When I was in St Michael's College, Llandaff, training for Ordination we observed a strict Holy Week regime. From Maundy Thursday at a certain point in the service the organ was turned off and we couldn't sing. Then on Easter Sunday at another certain point in the service the organ was switched on again, we made a joyful noise and we could sing again, this was such a moving experience. I can only imagine what it will be like when we can sing again in church, what joy there will be then. I am already excited at the prospect even though it seems such a long way off. Today is here now and it is today that we have to make the most of.

Have a good day today.

Kingsley

Tue 10 Nov

Dear Friends

Sitting here in my study looking out across the valley with the Roman Road passing in front of the Vicarage and all the people walking past I always felt I was in a goldfish bowl. Until it was pointed out that from the Roman Road you cannot see in, all you can see is the sky reflected on the windows. Only all of you who receive these emails can see into my inner self as I have been reflecting not the sky but my own thoughts. By now there can be very little you don't know about me, except odd things like the time I worked on road building sites with a pick and shovel. I now have to start thinking about Sundays again, I will have to prepare for Advent and Christmas, the Church year is going to push me along again. Whatever else this year with all its hardship, loss and sadness has given us all a new perspective and I have learned a lot about all those who have responded to these emails.

How much of ourselves do we ever truly reveal to others? There will always be those who reveal nothing but a public face and though they don't know it they are the losers for staying closed. Because opening up gives greater freedom, greater understanding of one another. We are meant to be social animals after all and the Bible is all about loving one another. Do not shut everyone out. Be yourselves not the person you want people to believe you are.

Kingsley

Wed 11 Nov

Dear Friends

During a long pilgrimage the pilgrims would tell each other stories to keep their spirits up especially on difficult patches. Stories that would have been passed on and very rarely written down, our myths and legends come from such stories which the church would have frowned on and modern people simply dismissed, but does that mean they were not true or at the very least based in truth? There is the famous story from Myddfai, a boy grazing sheep by a lake was dumbstruck when a beautiful lady emerged from the lake and promised him wealth and prosperity, they married and he prospered. However he was told she would return if he struck her three times, over the course of many years he did just that and she returned to the lake with all his cattle, sheep ducks etc. Later one of his sons met her and she gave him medical prescriptions and instructions and the doctors of Myddfai became renowned throughout the land and this is a matter of history.

There is more going on around us than we can possibly know, there is magic if we are willing to accept it.

Have a magical day

Kingsley

Thu 12 Nov

Dear Friends

With news of a vaccine and the possibility or normality in the spring things begin to look hopeful. But Jo-an and I were talking last night about the affect this will all have to very young children in years to come. The fear that has been installed in everyone, there is the news of so many deaths, they cannot hug their grandparents and everyone going around with masks, what is this doing to impressionable minds?

Which is all the more reason for us adults to have a positive outlook, especially around children. We should not give in to fear and we should keep as positive as possible. It is hard and for some people they have had a real struggle themselves. But it is important for those of us who can to remain cheerful.

We have a winter to get through before the spring and the new hope. When the first hunter gatherers came to this valley the winters were still hard, it was not long after the last ice age, they had to store as much food as they could, they had to huddle together and keep the fires burning. But they saw the winter through and they settled and in time the community thrived and grew. It is amazing how resilient human beings are, we can find a way, we can get through the hard times and we can thrive. From our perspective now this has been and still is a long hard drag but the spring is not far away. Even in the winter the first settlers found moments to celebrate and we have had our celebrations too. Trust in yourself, enjoy the moments and look forward with hope.

Kingsley

Fri 13 Nov

Dear Friends

In Wales we are preparing to go back to church on Sunday and I have every sympathy for those in England who can't. Going to church is not seen as essential and in a sense it isn't because we can pray anywhere. But it is more than just praying, it is a discipline - we are disciples after all - it is also a social gathering. Too many people have been cut off and isolated during this pandemic and the effects on mental health will have long term repercussions. Too many people have been separated from loved ones in homes and hospitals, unable to hold the hand of the dying. This is not a criticism of anyone because no one can possibly know what the best course of action is. I have said before that the future is an 'undiscovered country' and at no time has this been so obvious than now. Everyone, even the experts, were finding their way in the dark. At least now there is a better understanding, there are better treatments, there is more light, there is a vaccine, there is more hope.

So we can begin to plan again. We can have some idea of what we are going to do for Christmas and we are promised normality in the spring. I have been in touch with the Bishop and the Dean of the Cathedral both of whom are keen for us to have a celebration service in the Cathedral to mark the end of our pilgrimage. We may not have a date but at least we have a destination, I know it will not be possible for some of you to get there but you can be there in spirit. This may not have been a physical pilgrimage but it will have a physical end. There may be difficulties yet but an end is in sight.

When Mike, Sue and I were walking the Pembrokeshire Costal Path down steps and up steps, round yet another headland, there were times we thought we would never get there. But we did, and we have the certificates to prove it. Journeys do have an end, and don't forget journeys have plenty of joys along the way.

Kingsley

Sat 14 Nov

Dear Friends

We must continue to be vigilant. Now is not the time to let our guard down. We have come this far and although there are difficult times ahead we know there will be an end, we will get some sort of normality back, so press on.

The whole of life is a journey, it is a series of discoveries and new experiences. When I take a funeral I often comment that it is not the number of times the earth has circled the sun that is important, it is what we have filled our time with, our relationships with others and the effect we have had on others that really counts. Which is why the question 'how old was he/she' is such a stupid question. Some people manage to fill every moment of a short life while others can have very little to show for a long one. Life is not about talking about what you will one day do but about getting on and doing it. Spontaneity is a good thing, it may get you into scrapes but you will learn something from that too. Better than to sit and plan and allow the time to pass safely without doing. Today is another day full of hope and possibilities, use it.

Kingsley

Sun 15 Nov

Subject: Kingdom 3

Dear Friends

Matthew 25. 14-30. A man goes on a journey and gives three servants talents to look after while he is gone. The one he gives five to makes five more and the one he give two to makes two more. They are both commended and given extra responsibilities. The third is only given one which he buries and digs it up again when his master returns with the excuse that the master was hard and would reap what he hadn't sown, so his talent was taken from him and given to the one with ten and he was thrown out. This third servant had made an assumption about the master which was evidently not true because the two who had doubled their talents got to keep them as well as being given more responsibilities.

With every parable Jesus told it was only a part of what he was telling us not the whole. This parable tells us that God has given us a part to play, no matter how small, in building his kingdom. He does expect us to work but not for his benefit, rather for ours. We cannot sit back and expect God to do everything for us, such is the trust he put in us that we work with him and if our work is genuine he will work with us. He doesn't always tell us what to do, he doesn't need to, he knows we are quite capable ourselves. He believes in us, so let us play our part.

Kingsley

Mon 16 Nov

Subject: Week 34

Dear Friends

When it isn't overcast I live in a wonderful spot for stargazing, Mars is very bright in the sky at the moment.

My only problem is that my telescope is so heavy it is a bit of a struggle taking it out to have proper look. But that doesn't stop me pausing for a moment to look up into the skies at all the familiar constellations and ponder the vastness of space. When I was young I wanted to be an astronaut but there was very little opportunity to fulfil that dream, now I realise it was actually impossible because I suffer occasionally from vestibular neuritis, I do not have the balance for it. Still, one can dream. On this ball where we live we are still hurtling through space and if we can in our minds eye perceive just how small we are it should lead us on to some very profound questions. Questions about existence itself.

Yet here we are, going about our lives. And we are important, we are irreplaceable. What makes this true? God, The Maker Of All Things, who made the infinite vastness of the universe, cares for us all as individuals. I know this still leaves many questions unanswered, questions about suffering and loss. But the lonely, the outcast, the life too short to count would have no meaning at all in a Godless universe. No matter what, I find I have to believe in God, a God who will one day wipe the tears from our eyes because I cannot accept a universe where a stillborn child is not loved, a child who has their childhood ruined cannot have hope. Every life does count, every person is important, we all add something to this world.

Kingsley

Tue 17 Nov

Dear Friends

Looking out of my window today there are few leaves left on the trees, the sky is grey, the rain is falling, I cannot see the hills the other side of the valley. That is not what is bothering me, it is the prospect of two zoom meetings! I am not a meeting person but at least in a real meeting you can chat with one another. In a zoom meeting you must take your turn. Ah well, I might still learn something useful, I might get some news. I will look for the silver lining.

I miss the freedom of just going to someone's house, being invited in to have a chat and a cup of tea or coffee. This is one of the things that will indicate normality again when it happens, this freedom to visit. Other things will be the lack of tape all over the place, seeing people's faces without masks and singing. This will all come. However, no matter how depressing zoom meetings are I am going to look for something good today, I am still going to enjoy myself. And I wish you all happiness and joy today.

Kingsley

Wed 18 Nov

Dear Friends

My first experience of a computer was when I changed schools because the one I was in wasn't doing the

A levels I wanted to do, the new school had just dismantled their old computer which filled a room and now they shared a desktop computer with two other schools. And when I say desktop I mean something four times the size of a microwave oven that could be moved and stood on a desk, and even then you had to use a separate machine for typing out the punch tape in BASIC that you then had to feed into the computer and wait for the paper to come out with the answer. Now I have a device with far greater computing power quite apart from the multitude of other things it does in my pocket. The pace of technological change is mind blowing.

With Christmas coming up I will still be writing cards. My handwriting may be rubbish so on most occasions I type letters but sometimes it is worth making the effort to write legibly, it is more personal. One of the hardest things during this pandemic has been the restrictions of actually physically meeting with people apart from queueing up outside shops, and it is wonderful that we can meet up in Church, but even so we cannot sit down over a cup of tea and have a proper chat. Yes, technology has been wonderful during this time but I hope it hasn't changed things for ever, that we will get back our real lives. I hope we will not face the world through a screen just because it is convenient but we will make the effort to switch it off and go out and mix and visit.

Kingsley

Thu 19 Nov

Dear Friends

We have come such a long way since March, we haven't sat still and this has been such a time for learning for all of us. Many of us have learned new technologies (some of us are still struggling with it), we have learned much about ourselves and perhaps much about others which has surprised us in so many ways. There has been much sadness but there has been joy too. Our perspectives have changed, we have a better idea of what is important and what is not. We appreciate the simple things more. You will be interested to know that we can sing outside, if only we could be sure of the weather we could arrange to have an outdoor carol service.

I am planning for Advent and Christmas, I brought Jo-an's tree down from the loft and put it up in her sitting room yesterday, I am required to celebrate Communion at Christmas so the 11.30 Midnight service in St Mary's will be a half Communion service, bread only, and I need to work out how to do this considering the restrictions. I cannot have another service in the same church Christmas Day. We have to think through everything we do at the moment and it seems I am not the only one who feels like this, a lot of people I meet queueing up outside the paper shop say the same. Think through these things we do and we get on with life.

Plan ahead and look after yourselves.

Kingsley

Part 5
Brief Respite

Fri 20 Nov

Dear Friends

What a difference in two days. Today it is teeming with rain, a total contrast to yesterday. Yesterday I drove over to St Cledwyn's Church, Llanglydwen to go through the requirements to open the church with the Wardens. Can I have permission from the LMA please. It was a lovely drive through the countryside, with the Preseli Mountains clear as anything in the background, up and down country lanes through mile after mile of farmland, through Cefn Y Pant which I always refer to as the Back of Beyond, over the narrow bridge in Llanglydwen and up to surely one of the most grand entrances to a church anywhere and down to the lane to the church. Every church that opens is a sign to the community that even in the midst of the pandemic life is returning and the church survives. And the one thing that stands out, something I have always believed anyway, is that the church is the people who care for and look after the building where they meet for worship and are there for the community.

Even in our present difficulties there is life everywhere, the spring flowers wait just below the surface, the buds on the bare trees are preparing for new leaves, people everywhere are getting on with living and planning for the future. Pandora's box is open.

Every blessing

Kingsley

Sat 21 Nov

Dear Friends

It seems we are not the only ones decorating early for Christmas, North Road is lit all the way down. Amid all the gloom and worry people everywhere are determined to celebrate and make a show, and good for them. It is well known that during WWI the opposing armies in the trenches played football together at Christmas. The human spirit cannot be quenched and even in the ruin of war people will find time for good. The times we live in are sad, there is suffering, and there will be years of hardship ahead and we will still find opportunities to rejoice.

This is not me trying to cheer everyone up, this is what I see all around, this is people everywhere. This is also a time when you see so much good in people, those who put themselves out to do something for the lonely. So we rejoice also in the kindness of people.

Peace be with you.

Kingsley

Sun 22 Nov

Subject: Christ the King

Dear Friends

Matthew 25: 31-46. The warning of the sheep and the goats, the sheep being the people who have seen the need in others and helped them and in helping them have helped Jesus and therefore inherit their place in the kingdom, while the goats saw the need and did nothing and are cast out. This is a sobering passage but it is not a passage that people base the way they live on. The people who do not help others have taken no notice of it, this is just the way they are. While on the other hand the kind, the generous and helpful people are not that way out of fear of the warning but simply because of the goodness within that compels them to go out of their way to help others. This passage is not so much a warning but a statement. And it seems true of so much of the Bible, people will do the things they do because of who they are rather than what they have read. Fortunately there is far more goodness and kindness in this world, even though there is no one who is completely good and no one is completely bad.

This present pandemic is a testing time, it has highlighted who are sheep and who are goats, but it has shown how caring and thoughtful and kind so many people are certainly in communities like ours. Be a sheep today and not a goat.

Kingsley

Mon 23 Nov

Subject: Week 35

Dear Friends

Wonder of wonders, all four parts of the UK are in agreement, we can have Christmas! Four households will be able to meet together but they tell us there will have to be stricter measures afterwards. Meanwhile churches are preparing by finding ways of doing carol services without singing, communion without wine, doing the best we can. We will celebrate the Birth of Christ, God coming into the world, and this will be a bright light in the darkness. We need this because it has been a hard year, and as we move forward into the new year, the new spring, the lengthening of days let us draw strength from this time of hope and joy. The journey may not be over but we can rest along the way.

Rest awhile, rejoice, and press forward, rise up with wings as eagles, renew your resolve.

Kingsley

Tue 24 Nov

Dear Friends

I am reminded that clergy are entitled to take a sabbatical every ten years, which means I am overdue for mine and the church owes me six months. But what do clergy do with a sabbatical? Reflection, prayer and spiritual renewal, and maybe even write a book. Oh, I have been doing all that anyway as you all know, which is just as well because there isn't anyone to take my place if I did take the time off. This isn't to say I am indispensable because one day I will have to retire and the Church in Wales is not going to let the shiny new Ficerdy lie empty for long. But now is not the time. And what about all the lay people who have kept their churches going, who have done shopping for neighbours, who have helped in their communities, do they get a sabbatical?

I remember at the beginning of the first lockdown people were saying we are all in this together. And throughout my daily reflections I have felt closer to you in a strange way, I am so grateful to the people who have opened their churches and taken the services themselves, and I cannot put myself on a pedestal, I cannot set myself apart simply because I was ordained. This is why I would feel uncomfortable in a pulpit, and why I would not be happy with having wine at communion and not giving it to the congregation.

With the prospect of a vaccine and normality returning next year it will not be as it was, I have changed, the church has changed. I have reflected, I have prayed and I have been spiritually renewed and even written a book. Things will not be easy for a long time but there is a new world coming.

Kingsley

Wed 25 Nov

Dear Friends

Me, "Alexa, what is the meaning of life?" Alexa, "The answer is forty two but the question is more complicated."

Because humans are self-aware we can ask questions like this, probably the vast majority of people don't. Sometimes I think my life would be a lot simpler if I didn't and stuck to "What's for dinner?" but instead I have a mind that is always asking questions. One that bothers me is "How would I feel if I didn't exist?" another is "Why does anything exist?" I can see a few of you jumping up and down now shouting at your screen, "God made existence" without explaining why God exists in the first place. Ah, I think I'll stick with "What's for dinner?"

Existence does exist and it is good to pause a while and marvel at it all, from the vastness of space and the whirling of galaxies, stars, planets, down to the fragile spring flowers waiting in the hard earth to burst forth early next year and the drop of dew on the spiders web sparkling a little rainbow in the sunlight. And us somewhere in between that God has given eyes to that we may see and an appreciation that we may marvel. And for all the sadness in the world the universe is a place of endless wonder.

Open your eyes to wonder today

Kingsley

Thu 26 Nov

Dear Friends

It is a cold and frosty morning and the mist is so thick I can only see half way down to Whitland. The changing of the seasons, the variations in the weather from day to day add to the experience of life. We continue to live from day to day and slowly the world turns and orbits the sun. For us in the northern hemisphere the tilt of the earth turns us somewhat away from the sun and in less than a month we will have the shortest day and the cycle begins again.

In one way this has been a lost year because of all the things we haven't been able to do. Yet in another way it has been such a long year and we have had the opportunity to reflect on what is important, we have had to reassess everything. As we enter Advent on Sunday we must take time to examine ourselves and our relationship with God and with one another. Advent, like Lent, is supposed to be a preparation, although it is the run up to Christmas it always has the double meaning of Jesus return at the end of the world and we must be sure we are prepared for him should this be the time he comes. Could we face him and say we have done all we should?

Yet Christmas is the time when we rejoice that God came into the world because he cares for us personally and he knows we are not perfect and he accepts us even so.

Kingsley

Fri 27 Nov

Dear Friends

I am off to Llanwinio this afternoon to risk assess another church for opening, do I have the LMA's permission?

Can you keep a secret? People like to know a secret that others don't but some people are better at keeping secrets than others. If I want everyone to know a secret I know the very people to tell it to. However if I want a secret kept I know who will keep it. Yet the best place for a secret is hidden in plain sight, for some reason people can't see it even if you tell them there is one. Everyone knows there is one in my book but no one has found it.

The secret of the Kingdom, of eternal life, is just such a secret. It is in plain sight, it runs through the Bible, it is being shouted in nature all the time. And yet so many people do not see it possibly because they are afraid of the cost, they will have to give something up, they will be asked to do something by God. Christmas is a time when this secret is made blatantly obvious, 'God so loved the world that he sent his only Son.' The secret is that God is not remote, he is standing at the door of our hearts knocking to be let in, and the only demand he makes is that we love him and love one another.

Knock knock

Kingsley

Sat 28 Nov

Dear Friends

With further restrictions again from next Friday in Wales and most of England in Tier 3 things are looking bleak. I won't know for a few days where the churches are in all this. This is another hard stretch of our journey, so we gather our cloaks around us against the storms and press on. Perhaps at times like this the pilgrims of old would begin to sing or tell stories to lift their spirits. A journey with others is always better than a journey alone and we know we take this journey together and it is not only through modern technology that we are in touch with one another but in spirit too.

Don't give up now, we have already come so far. Now is the time to hold on to your dreams and hopes and know there are better times ahead. Love 'always protects, always trusts, always hopes, always perseveres.' The human spirit it always greater than sometimes we realise because it is the likeness of God in us.

Kingsley

Part 6
Advent

Sun 29 Nov

Subject: The First Sunday of Advent

Dear Friends

In the new lectionary the gospel reading is Mark 13. 24-37, signs of the end of the age and a reminder to keep alert because we don't know when Jesus will return. While in the 1984 Church in Wales book the gospel is Matthew 21. 1-13, Jesus entry into Jerusalem and overturning the stalls in the temple. Certainly not the little Jesus meek and mild safely tucked up in the manger. Advent is a time to prepare for his coming and it will not be what we expect, he will overturn many of our preconceptions, are we truly ready for him? We may or may not be living in the last days but this much is certain we will have to face him some time. Whatever we think we have done we cannot work our own passage into heaven.

Praise be to God it is not on our own merits that we have eternal life but by his mercy. This is why he came to Earth all those years ago in Bethlehem, to live the example we must try to follow, to die on our behalf and to break the bonds of death for us. Christmas is a celebration not simply because it is his birthday but because God entered our world. And we need to be aware that if God enters our own personal world he will turn it upside down. In Advent let us prepare our hearts to have our lives turned upside down.

Kingsley

Mon 30 Nov

Subject: Week 36

Dear Friends

Yesterday was very misty here, the visibility wasn't very far. In the afternoon we decided to drive to Amroth to walk along the front, when we got out of the valley it was bright sunshine. We watched the sun go down in a glory of colour over the sea and when it started getting cold we returned. As we got to the top of the hill overlooking Whitland the whole valley was filled with mist like the sea and we drove back down into it.

Sometimes we cannot see very far, everything is unclear. Above the mist of life the sun is shining if only we can rise above our present uncertainty. This is where faith comes in. In our spirit we can bask in the sunlight and see the glories beyond.

Kingsley

Tue 1 Dec

Dear Friends

With all the other restrictions the Church has not been compelled to close this time, and in the Archdeacon's Bulletin this morning he points out that as larger family gatherings will be allowed for Christmas they can sit together in Church which raises our capacity. So some good news. Moreover we have rolled through space into December and here the sun is shining. I continue to pray for those of you who are under stricter restrictions and for all who still suffer or are lonely.

In today's gospel reading Jesus seems to be in a particularly good mood (Luke 10. 21-24). Sometimes people think he is a character in a story, but he was a real human being who lived the same as we do, he had good days and bad days. It would have been no good if he had just drifted through his life as if he was somehow out of it, he was fully immersed in life. His followers were lucky, they were with him in person, we have to rely on what is written in the Bible and whatever experiences we have through faith. We have so many questions, but even if he was here he would probably only answer with another question. This isn't because he is being deliberately awkward but because he trusts us to find out ourselves. Time for us to trust ourselves.

Kingsley

Wed 2 Dec

Dear Friends

To open up your soul, to let people into your life, your heart, means you will get hurt. People who you trust can let you down. So what can you do? You can shut yourself away, you can close the doors to those around you, you can trust no one but yourself, but you become lonely and isolated. Or you can continue to trust because no one is perfect not even yourself. You can continue to open your heart because the benefits are so much greater. You can look for the good in people because it is there somewhere. Then you will learn who you can trust and who you can't, if you close yourself up you will never find the people who you can trust. If you view everyone with suspicion you have already judged and condemned. But in reality, for all peoples faults, there is so much more good in this world, there is so much more good in people. If you were afraid of being run over by a car you would never go outside, if you were afraid of falling over you would never walk. Do not be afraid of trusting because despite the dangers there is so much to gain.

I have put a lot of trust in these emails, I have opened my heart and my soul, and the responses I have had have been wonderful and uplifting, some of you have opened your souls to me too. For all that I hate technology this has been a bright thread throughout the pandemic and I for one am richer for it.

Kingsley

Thu 3 Dec

Dear Friends

The pandemic and the lockdowns and the restrictions have affected us all in so many ways and not all of them obvious. We have lost a way of life, we have lost so many freedoms, it is bound to affect us all deeply. There are those who claim this is some sort of judgement but it isn't, because the poor and the vulnerable are worst affected while the rich seem to be sailing above safely tucked away in ivory towers. It has highlighted the selfish and greedy on the one hand and the good and selfless on the other but we knew who was who anyway and didn't need it highlighted. If anything this is a result of humans tampering with nature, and to the question of why God has allowed this I still have no answer.

There was never a promise that life was going to be easy, only that God would be with us. He didn't make it easy for his Son. Still there are so many good things in life that more than compensate for the bad, the world itself is such a beautiful place and the wonders of nature are all around, and the human spirit will smile. There is still magic, if only I had a magic wand ... I just remembered I have so here I am waving it.

Expect magic today.

Kingsley

Fri 4 Dec

Dear Friends

With the vaccine beginning to be administered and the promise of normality in the spring I'm sure we can manage through some possibly difficult times this winter. Some parts of the country have already had snow but at the moment here it is bright and sunny and bitterly cold.

Every season has charm, even winter with its shorter days has its highlights. Not long now and we will pass the shortest day and we will celebrate Christmas, though there is still a lot of winter to get through after that. But we will have turned the corner. The journey is not yet over but we begin to realise there is an end. Do not just look forward to the brighter future, make the most of now, enjoy each today for what it brings. Wrap up warm and keep safe.

Kingsley

Sat 5 Dec

Dear Friends

Please bear with me while I try to explain something I don't think I can explain. In the Lord of the Rings while in Lothlorien Sam follows Frodo and Galadriel, apart from anything else Sam wants to see magic, Galadriel knows what Sam means but doesn't see it as magic herself because it is just part of the nature of the place itself where she is the guardian. In my travels, first as Area Dean of South Pembrokeshire and now as Ministry Area Dean of East Landsker, I find there is a magic of place, you might call it spirit, and each place is different. So much of West Wales is unspoilt and therefore the different feel of places is perhaps more obvious. My joy and privilege is to go to different places to the churches and in the quiet of the countryside to experience the magic of place. Everyone knows about places like Iona and Lindisfarne but this is everywhere. Obviously I am more aware of this where I live and I have found the same spirit from Cyffig to Llanddewi Velfy to Llanboidy. God often reaches us through the quiet and the peace, when we are still enough to listen, in the still small voice.

Be still and know that I am God

So be still today, if only for a moment, and just be in the presence of God.

Kingsley

Sun 6 Dec

Subject: The Second Sunday of Advent

Dear Friends

Mark 1. 1-8. Mark launches straight into John the Baptist fulfilling the prophecy of Isaiah preparing the way for the Lord and the people flocking out to the desert to hear him and be baptised. There is no explanation as to who he is, and in the next verse Jesus turns up to be baptised too. If this had been the only gospel we would have been left to guess what was going on. But Mark was writing to people who knew, it was written to encourage the church in the face of persecution. I always feel for John the Baptist. He went out into the desert at an early age and survived the best he could, he hadn't long began his ministry which had a great impact until Jesus came along and eclipsed him, later he was arrested, imprisoned and beheaded. The life of a prophet was tough and those who God speaks through don't seem to have a choice. So many people in the world don't want to hear the truth.

And yet the truth is life and peace and joy and hope, what could possibly be wrong with that? What can greedy, selfish, nasty and cruel people possibly get out of being like that?

John came to prepare the way, to turn the hearts of people away from sin, to announce the arrival of the Messiah. This Advent let us prepare our hearts again for his coming, let us open up our lives to receive Jesus.

Kingsley

Mon 7 Dec

Subject: Week 37

Dear Friends

Now is a time of mixed feelings. There is a vaccine and injections start this week but it will take a long time to get to everyone, we rejoice that there will be greater freedom for Christmas but will we have to pay for it in January? We can only do what we have done throughout the pandemic. Listen to advice, be careful in everything we do, and continue to live every day as it comes. Time passes so quickly we should not wish our lives away impatient for a brighter future. Besides which when things return to some sort of normality we cannot escape the fact that it will not be as it was, so much has changed, we are going through traumatic times and we will not be able to wipe all that out as if it never happened. Don't expect the church to be the same either, I will have to review the services I can take at least until we know what is happening with vacancies.

But now is now, and all the churches that are open are doing very well thanks to the people of the churches themselves. We continue to prepare our hearts through Advent for the coming of Jesus. We take time to be quiet and listen. We support one another. We look for the magic in each day and the joys it holds. (For those of you who read this in the evening then this goes for tomorrow). Pray for peace, pray for healing, pray for hope.

Kingsley

Tue 8 Dec

Dear Friends

Despite the fact that all this began in March, that I have been writing these daily emails almost from the beginning, that I have helped tape up pews in many churches and filled in many risk assessment forms, I still don't think I have really come to terms with what has happened. I have had a chance to reflect, to pray, to question, but life has been so strange at times it doesn't seem real. I have often written about what is normal because normal changes all the time and the normal of the past has gone, the normal of the future is unknown and we live in the normal of now.

We are so fortunate here that we are having a spell of bright sunny weather with cold and frosty mornings, the sort of winter I really like. The world of nature around us is unaffected and the earth is spinning round the sun and bringing us the seasons, the leaves have fallen from the trees and wait to bud again, the soil hides the new growth to burst forth in the spring, the sheep will soon be lambing and keeping the farmers very busy, I have already seen primroses. We human beings are only visiting, if only we took time to appreciate what is around us rather than thinking we are the centre of all things. God has given us such beauty, as we approach Christmas we remember that he has given us such a promise of hope and joy, let us look beyond ourselves.

Kingsley

Wed 9 Dec

Subject: Still reflecting

Dear Friends

Those of you who have been with me from the beginning and those who have read the book will know, although the lockdown began on 23rd March my first email was 25th just to keep in touch, the next was 3rd April. This started to be a daily email on Palm Sunday 5th Apr and it was at your request that I continued after Easter. Therefore 5th of April will be the anniversary, I have now got a date for you to pencil in to your diaries, Saturday 10th April 2021, 3.00 pm, Meeting in St David's Shrine followed by a service in St David's Cathedral. We do not know what the state of things will be by then but I felt it was important to set a date as close to the anniversary as possible. This is still four months off and there is still so much of the journey to go through, and the journey itself in many ways is more important than the destination.

We have learned much from each other and I am enjoying your company. I hope you realise that the days when the Vicar did everything has gone and you have found you are just as important for the church and for the kingdom. This pilgrimage has been about all of us. I trust we have all found ourselves, if not there is still time. If there is a vision for the future of the church it is not in the clergy but in every Christian.

God bless you all today.

Kingsley

Thu 10 Dec

Dear Friends

Major events have always changed the world, or rather the lives of the people who live in it, usually it is the wars that have had the greatest impact. This pandemic has changed the world, or at least hurried on the changes that would inevitably happen anyway. The internet has taken over many things, from meetings where people no longer have to travel and gather together, to working from home, to shopping on line. I was talking to the postman the other day he said he has been so very busy he is always running late because of the packages he has to deliver, but he is getting used to it. One thing that was becoming the latest thing before the pandemic which seems to have been forgotten about is face recognition technology, what is the use when everyone wears masks.

And, of course, as I mentioned recently the church has changed. We no longer have the vestiges of a Victorian Church apart from one or two people who think we still live there. Christianity would not have spread so rapidly in the early days if the Romans had not destroyed much of Jerusalem including the Temple and forced the church out of their comfort zone into the world. This pandemic has shown us that Christianity is more than the buildings and the Vicar. It is up to all of us to make the church what we need and what the world needs. A new world is open before us, let us make the most of it.

Kingsley

Fri 11 Dec

Dear Friends

The publishers of the book sent a copy to The British Library, The Bodleian Library of Oxford, The

Cambridge University Library, The National Library of Scotland, The Library of Trinity College Dublin and the National Library of Wales in Aberystwyth. Little did I realise when I began these emails that they would be recorded for posterity and perhaps some future historian will look back at them to see what it was like to live through this pandemic. And if these present emails are also published it is a sobering thought that when I press the SEND I commit my ramblings to history. So does this make a difference to what I say? Not at all, I still think of all of you as I tap away, of what we are going through together, our fears and hopes, our joys and sorrows. I find this is still a personal journey with you as friends and from time to time I will reveal a little more about myself.

As we continue through Advent we must remember it is a time of preparation, we are preparing for God, The Maker Of All Things, to enter our world and our hearts. Jesus is standing at the door and knocking, are we ready to let him in? We do not have to be perfect, we do not need to sweep the floors and fluff up the cushions, he will come in and accept us as we are. All he is concerned with is the welcome.

Kingsley

Sat 12 Dec

Dear Friends

With the threat of a possible lockdown after Christmas, or at least stricter rules, it makes me wonder do people make too much of Christmas without realising what we are really celebrating? Surely a simple Christmas is all we need. But I suppose the government are bowing to the inevitable in that people will go overboard anyway and you can't fine everyone. It is worth noting that the early Church didn't make much of Christmas at all, Easter was the important celebration for them. It could be argued that we only started celebrating Christmas in this part of the world because the church wanted to Christianise the Winter Solstice and I only recently found out that Christmas was originally on 21st December until the calendar was adjusted.

Be that as it may. I have often pointed out that pre-Christian is not pre-God, that the ancient people were trying to make sense of the world they lived in and powers greater than themselves and I see nothing wrong with celebrating the return of the sun and light into a dark world as a sign that God put in place before he entered the World as Jesus at Bethlehem. He is The Maker Of All Things and the whole of nature points to him. God incarnate is the centre of history, both before and after, it was always his intention as the only way to save us. Christmas is not a time to over indulge but a time of light and hope. Christmas is a time to put darkness behind us and open ourselves to the light.

Oops, I think I have just preached my Christmas sermon! I'll have to think of something else now.

Kingsley

Sun 13 Dec

Subject: The Third Sunday of Advent

Dear Friends

John 1. 6-8, 19-28. John the Baptist was sent by God to be a witness to the light and he humbly accepted his role, he had no pretention to be anything more, and when questioned would only admit to being the fulfilment of the prophecy of the voice in the wilderness. This is such a rare quality, anyone else seeing the people flocking out to hear him and be baptised by him would have been swayed into thinking they were important. But he knew he was simply the messenger and the message was what was important. Sadly throughout the history of the church the message has been secondary at times to all the pomp and show and self-importance of people with titles. And yet, at heart the message has remained always through the simple honesty of the ordinary people, if anyone can be called ordinary. When it comes to spreading the message it is in the daily lives of people living in the world, through their example as they suffer the same tragedies as those around them, the same joys, the same worries and the same hopes. We are the voices in the wilderness, we are the bearers of the message and it is through what we do in our communities that the message is spread. We do not need eloquent words we just need to be and the message of joy and hope and peace will shine through us.

Prepare the way for he is coming.

Kingsley

Mon 14 Dec

Subject: Week 38

Dear Friends

There was magic yesterday in St. Mary's. Mary our organist had suggested we have a nine lessons and carols but that she would play a verse of each carol we would have sung in between the readings so this is what we did, this was special in itself but what was truly magical was when the angels and shepherds turned up and read the lesson of the angels and the shepherds thanks to Janine's family. My thanks to all who read too it was good to hear other voices than mine both in Whitland and in Cyffig in the afternoon. In the depths of the pandemic there is still joy, we are doing our best to rise above our present situation.

After all Christmas is all about the light shining in the darkness. In a dark room it only takes one candle and the room is no longer dark. Be that candle wherever you are.

Kingsley

Tue 15 Dec

Subject: Still shining (From today onwards I replace Still reflecting with Still shining because yesterday I spoke of a light shining in the darkness.)

Dear Friends

I had a very surreal event on Monday. For some days I have had a niggly headache, slight dizziness and nausea which is usually due to my inner ear, but I thought it would be advisable to have a COVID-19 test just to be sure, at first they wouldn't do it until I said I had a slight temperature. Driving round the Carmarthen showground from Hi-Viz jacketed people in huts between cones to other Hi-Viz jacketed people in huts I felt I was in some sort of post-apocalypse film, it was really quite creepy. You will be pleased to know I tested negative. But more and more it seems we are living in a different world. With the rules for Christmas now in doubt it is not surprising people are feeling the strain. We are very much living from day to day, one foot in front of another along our journey.

The rules might change for Christmas but it is still going to happen, we will still celebrate even if on a smaller scale. Even if Herod would cause devastation in Bethlehem after Jesus' birth the angels still sang to the shepherds who went to the stable with joy, the Magi still travelled a great distance to see the wonder of God come to earth. And one day we will enter the green phase, one day we will sing, one day we will cwtch. One day we will be able to look back and be proud of how we coped. One day the world will be free again. Hold on.

Kingsley

Part 7
Reduced Christmas

Thu 17 Dec

Dear Friends

So now we know, in Wales Christmas gatherings are limited to two households and from 28th December back into lockdown. One of the differences with this third lockdown is that places of worship can still hold services.

I have noticed a difference in people and in the general atmosphere. People are less cheerful, the worry and the changing rules and the length of time is all wearing everyone down. I promise you all that I will remain cheerful and continue to look on the bright side.

As we work our way through Advent and approach Christmas it is significant that an event is happening in the sky that is rare, it last happened 800 years ago. Jupiter and Saturn are coming together from our perspective and people are saying this is the star of Bethlehem. In the middle of this dark and frightening time the star has returned to renew our hope, the promise of light. A sign in the sky to lead us to the stable and see the wonder of God born in human form.

Perhaps because we cannot sing we will hear the angels sing instead. We are forced to keep silent so the whole of nature will shout. This Christmas will be different but let us make it special.

Kingsley

Fri 18 Dec

Dear Friends

Legend has it that Mary and Joseph travelled for five days from Nazareth to Bethlehem, so today they are packing up and getting ready for the journey. I have often wondered why just them? Didn't they have family who would also have been descended from David? If, as Catholics claim, the mention of Jesus brothers in the Bible are half-brothers because Joseph had children by his first marriage and he was a widower where are they? Where are their cousins? Or was their journey to Bethlehem really such a lonely journey as is always depicted? There are so many things we are not told. If this was a simple story none of this would matter but it wasn't just a simple story, these were real people with real lives.

They had also been visited by angels. Real people with real lives visited by angels which means the angels are just as real, they are part of the world we live in though mostly unseen. Not everything in this world can be seen or proved and by discounting what you cannot see or prove you close your mind to the possibility of wonder and magic. Christmas is more than partying, more than getting together, it is celebrating the joining of heaven and earth, it is opening the door to endless wonder, it is opening our hearts to dreams and hopes.

Kingsley

Sat 19 Dec

Dear Friends

Mary and Joseph set out for Bethlehem, the Bible says practically nothing about this, only Matthew says that they did. So you will excuse me if I rely on tradition. This was a long journey and most people had to walk. Joseph, being a carpenter, could afford a donkey to carry enough provision for the journey. And because Mary was heavily pregnant she would have ridden much of the way. Possibly the easiest route would have been to make for the Jordan to travel down the valley, this would be fitting as the Jordan would feature later in Jesus' life. Throughout the journey Mary and Joseph would trust in God to keep them safe and protect the baby because of the messages from the angels, but they were still an ordinary little couple not endowed with divine powers, they had been asked by God to fulfil a purpose and since when has God actually made it easy? They still had to trudge along, and Mary in the state she was, they had to eat and rest along the way. Sometimes God expects so much from his faithful people.

We have been travelling this difficult path since March, so let us for a few days travel with Mary and Joseph rather than get caught up with all the hype because this year we have the time to reflect. God may expect much but he always gives so much more.

Kingsley

Sun 20 Dec

Subject: The Fourth Sunday of Advent

Dear Friends

Luke 1. 26-38. As Mary and Joseph journey to Bethlehem I expect there were times they got very weary, after all this is a journey they did not want to take, it was forced on them by the Romans. Mary is heavily pregnant and could give birth at any time. It would be at times like this that I am sure she would reflect back to the visit of the angel Gabriel. The visit of an angel is an amazing and daunting experience event in itself, but to be told you have found favour with God and are to bear His Son! This had kept her going through the difficult times of possibly losing Joseph and the chattering tongues of the neighbours and it would keep her going through this arduous journey. She had found favour with God and still God didn't make it easy for her.

Suddenly we are thrown back into lockdown, or tier 4 as they are calling it, a week early. This time the church can remain open but we all need to be extra careful. We face a very difficult stage of our journey and God isn't going to make it easy for us, but whatever vision or experience of him we had in our past or trust we have in the present will have to be enough to see us through. Also our own prayers and the support of one another. God hasn't brought us this far to abandon us and there is still hope in the future. In the meantime, as I have often said, the journey is an experience in itself and there are still things for us to learn from our own reflections and the friendship of those who travel with us. Each day is a gift, use it wisely.

Kingsley

Mon 21 Dec

Subject: Week 39

Dear Friends

I like the children's song 'Little Donkey' because in its simple way it reminds us it was not an easy journey but there would be such joy at the end. We can learn something about who Joseph and Mary were from snippets in the Bible. Joseph was a good and honest man, when he discovered Mary was pregnant he still wanted to protect her and when the angel visited him as well he was willing to fit in with God's plan. Mary was a humble quiet person, not wanting to make a fuss, we hear in Luke's Gospel of her treasuring things in her heart, I personally think she would not be too happy with the fuss the church has made of her. An ordinary couple being obedient to God. As they travel to Bethlehem we cannot imagine the mixture of feelings they are having, a simple couple with an extraordinary responsibility.

As we travel our journey we have a responsibility too, to spread joy and hope in these dark days. Jo-an and I went up the hill last night to look at the star of Bethlehem, that is the conjunction of Jupiter and Saturn, in case it would be too cloudy tonight. Sometimes we can be so busy looking down we forget to look up, now is the time to look up to see the wonders in the sky and glimpse the angels and hear them sing.

Kingsley

Tue 22 Dec

Dear Friends

Mary and Joseph are trudging south along the Jordan valley which is a fertile area between mountains, the Jordan flows down from the Sea of Galilee into the Dead Sea and is below sea level, and it is not an easy journey. When we recount the Christmas story it tends to be just that, a story, we need to take time to think where Mary and Joseph were each day, they are only half way through their journey and the more difficult part is yet to come and don't forget Mary is heavily pregnant and could give birth at any moment. When we get to Christmas remember what they had to go through, the sacrifice, the commitment, the obedience, so much more than a pretty story.

One day we will look back at our journey now and future generations will not know what it was like for us, we will tell them but it will not be the same as living through it. The fear, the worry, the anxiety, the tragedies, the heartache, the loss of a life that was. But let us not forget the good things too, the time we have to reflect on our lives, on what is important, finding God in so many places outside church, the goodness of communities and the generosity of people. Whatever the politicians and leaders do it is us who are living through this and making the most of what we have. Life has gone on, this is an experience that will be with us into the future, make it count.

Kingsley

Wed 23 Dec

Dear Friends

Today Mary and Joseph will come to the point that Joshua parted the Jordan and brought the people of Israel into the Promised Land, then they will make their way out of the valley up to Jericho where perhaps they will spend the night. History and tradition are important to the Jews so I am sure they will feel this is a special part of their journey, and at the same time Mary is bearing the fulfilment of prophecy and the hope of the future. But it is the road they are on that is most important, their weariness and present concerns.

Living in the now means we are always living in the point between the past and the future. The past is important because it has brought us to the point where we are, it has given us the basis for all we have learned and the future is the hope of tomorrow. But as always the present moment is where we are and what we do now is what is most important. Through this pandemic I have often said that the past is gone, our way of life has changed and the future new world is unknown. We are building the future now, and how we live now will determine what the world will be. We may feel powerless, fearful and anxious, but it is how deal with it that is our power to shape what is to come.

Let us build a better world.

Kingsley

Thu 24 Dec

Subject: Christmas Eve

Dear Friends

Today is the final part of the journey for Mary and Joseph. From Jericho up to Jerusalem and then across to Bethlehem, not a particularly safe route as the Samaritan found the man beaten and robbed between Jericho and Jerusalem. Fortunately as people were gathering for the census there would have been a good many traveling this road today. Mary and Joseph would have got to Bethlehem quite late in the day by which time all the available accommodation had been filled. We can excuse Joseph for being fraught with worry as he begged for somewhere to stay, and we can forgive Mary for being scared, she was only young having her first baby in a strange crowded place. And so someone took pity on this young couple and took them to the stable. For everyone else although they resented the orders of the Romans to be there they caught up with relatives they hadn't seen for a long time or perhaps not even met, I expect there was a lot of celebration going on. And quietly, unnoticed, Mary and Joseph settled in and prepared.

Tonight in St Mary's Church at 11.30 and in many churches all over the world some people will come away from their festivities for a moment to the quiet of a church and remember to praise God for bringing heaven and earth together. To hear the news again that God is born a human, not in a palace, not with the rich and famous, not with celebrities, not with the powerful, but a simple couple in a stable.

Kingsley

Fri 25 Dec

Subject: Christmas Day

Dear Friends

Christ is born, God with us, the heavens rejoice and all of nature too, we are given light in our darkness, hope in our despair, joy in our sadness. To Mary a Son, and she is given no peace as the shepherds burst in, and Joseph holds her hand, he still wants to protect her. No more are heaven and earth separate places, they are one even when we can't see it. And the simple couple are given the responsibility for God's humanity, they are at the turning point of all history.

We are at a turning point in history too though to a lesser extent. It is up to us to make something of today, we have the responsibility of the future, to make something good out of something bad, to be light in the dark world and to spread hope wherever we go. Make Christmas mean Christmas.

Happy Christmas.

Kingsley

Sat 26 Dec

Subject: Stephen, Deacon and First Martyr

Dear Friends

We will leave Mary and Joseph and their baby for a while so they can have a little peace. Stephen I have mentioned before in an earlier email. Wenceslaus I, Duke of Bohemia, King is quietly warming himself in front of an open fire and looking out of his window at the snow and you know the rest, but did you know he was assassinated in 935 and that his younger brother Boleslaus the Cruel was complicit? There is a real person with a real life behind even this heart-warming carol, and life can at times be hard and cruel, but people all over the world remember Wenseslaus and no one remembers his brother. Acts of kindness never go unnoticed.

After the brief respite of yesterday we again face an uncertain future and we trudge on through the present.

Yet as yonder peasant found there is always someone there to help and always from the most unexpected of people. As the Queen said in her speech yesterday (though actually is was the day before) this has brought us all closer together. And the message of Christmas, God himself coming into the world, there is the promise of light, a new dawn, even in the darkest of times. The shortest day is past but there is still a lot of winter to get through. We have lived through this pandemic since March, the journey we have ahead of us is shorter than behind us. The light is coming and we will rejoice again, we will sing and we will cwtch.

Kingsley

Sun 27 Dec

Subject: John, Apostle and Evangelist

Dear Friends

John 21. 19b-25. After the resurrection and Jesus reinstates Peter he turns to see John and asks Jesus, "Lord, what about him?" but John's role in the future is different to Peter's. He goes on to write the gospel that bears his name, he is exiled to Patmos where he has visions and writes the book Revelation and lives to an old age. Everyone has a different part to play and it is not up to us what God has called someone else to do, we each do our best with the gifts we are given. We are all important to the whole therefore there is no superiority or inferiority. None of us can look down on anyone else nor feel intimidated by others, we are equal in God's eyes. If only we realised this, the whole history of humanity would be so different.

As we approach the end of the year and 2021 beckons we know things are still going to be hard for some time, but we each have our part to play in helping and encouraging each other. God has entered the world, the darkness has no power, we live in the light let us be confident in this knowledge. Let us listen carefully to what God is asking each of us to do.

Kingsley

Mon 28 Dec

Subject: Week 40

Dear Friends

Mary and Joseph couldn't just wait around in the stable for people to visit, they couldn't live off fresh air or hand-outs. They couldn't undertake a journey back to Nazareth with a new baby. Surely Joseph would have looked for work and maybe have set up a carpentry business of his own, they would also have looked for somewhere more permanent to stay. Life for saints and holy people is exactly the same as for anyone else. Since God sent his Son to live a normal life then Mary and Joseph had to get on with the practicality of real life. There will be plenty of hardship to come.

Christmas has come and gone and we are in that strange period between Christmas and the New Year, we may not need to buy much food for a few days but there is still bread and milk to get. Many people are itching to say good riddance to 2020 but the beginning of 2021 isn't going to be much better. Storms and snow batter the country. So we get on with the practicality of living. As always we take one day at a time and each day has something new to bring us, round the next corner is something else we haven't seen, a new wonder, a new surprise. Each day holds promise so let us look for it. Let us live life to the full, even now.

Kingsley

Tue 29 Dec

Dear Friends

We all have hopes for the New Year, we all have dreams, despite the situation we are in now is still a good time to think about our hopes and dreams. We are coming out of the shorter days (except for those of you in Australia!) and although it is a while off yet Spring is on the way, nature is beginning to stir even if it is snowing or flooding. So too our hearts can stir, we can make our wishes, because although 2021 might not start well it is a year full of hope. Wishes rarely happen overnight, they will not come straight away on January 1st, like the flowers and the leaves slowly budding so will our hopes for the New Year. We must all be patient and all will be well. We have a few days left of 2020, let us use those days to set our sights on the brighter future while not forgetting to live in the present. And let us not write off 2020 as a total waste, so many good things have happened, we have all had to change the way we think and the way we look at the world and I hope we are all better people because of it.

Kingsley

Wed 30 Dec

Dear Friends

One of the things people say to me a lot is "I don't know how you find something different to say every day." And I am thinking to myself "Doesn't everyone?" I can't believe people say the same thing every day as if they are stuck in a loop. It may seem like it at times because this pandemic is dragging on but we are not stuck in a loop. Every day is a new day and it holds its own promise, every day is different.

When I worked for the Transport and Road Research Laboratory we would have students on a sandwich course working with us for a few months. One year we had students from China and one of them said to me "I know why you English talk about the weather so much, it is so interesting because it changes all the time."

But it is not just the weather that changes. The dynamics of the interaction of people changes, there is always some news in a community. The newspapers may seem like they are going over the same thing all the time but you can always find something different. There was a full moon last night and because we are people of this world it will affect us in some way for change. This is a world of infinite variety, endless wonder. Surely I am not the only one to find something different to say every day.

Kingsley

Thu 31 Dec

Subject: New Year's Eve

Dear Friends

The Old Year has almost run its course and this year will be remembered for a long time to come, the year when there was so much suffering and sadness, the year that shut practically everything down, the year that turned our lives upside down. But remember it was the year when we saw so much goodness in our local communities, the year when people were still able to get on with their lives through adversity, the year when so many people showed a dogged resilience. It was also a year when it showed what people were made of, the stupid and thoughtless, the lazy and selfish, but especially the good and kind and selfless, the heroes who kept things going. Do not write off the year because of what you could not do, accept the year for what it was, an opportunity for us to show our better side if we were willing, a year to reassess what is important, a year to reflect.

This has been a journey like no other and although it is not over we know there will be an end. I know people are very wary at the moment and the New Year will be welcomed in by most people quietly but it is still a milestone where we can look back at where we have come from and look forward with hope to where we are going. I want to thank everyone who has been on this journey with me, for your encouraging replies, for your friendship and the times I have been able to meet many of you in person and I wish you all a Happy New Year.

Kingsley

Part 8
2021

Fri 1 Jan

Subject: 2021

Dear Friends

It is only a short journey from Bethlehem to Jerusalem, less than 6 miles, and today we celebrate Mary and Joseph taking Jesus to the temple for his circumcision and naming ceremony. Here they meet Simeon who God had told would see the Messiah before he died, and Anna who spoke of the redemption of Jerusalem. This was the day that Jesus' birth was officially recorded at the temple, the setting in motion of events that would change the world.

Although there isn't a sign planted in space that the earth passes to say we have entered a New Year so to all intents and purposes it is a day like any other it still holds a special place in our human psyche. We make resolutions, we plan to make changes in our lives and I wonder if anyone actually keeps them for long. We always have hopes for the New Year, our hopes for the last New Year may have been dashed but events had already been set in motion that would change the world again. Events have been set in motion already for this year and it is worth hoping again. Over and over again people have said, me included, that we live in strange times, but that is just it - we live in time. We live each day for what it brings and each day is unknown until we live it, and after it becomes part of our experience, part of our life. The tapestry is woven and we can only see the picture when we look back. Take whatever today brings and treasure it. Today was a strange day for Mary and Joseph and some of the prophecies for them were not good but they still treasured the day.

I wish you health in body, mind and spirit this New Year.

Kingsley

Sat 2 Jan

Dear Friends

As we look at the universe, the stars in the galaxy, the orbits of the planets, we see balance everywhere. We see balance in the seasons, balance in the tides of the sea, balance in the natural world, balance among the animals. It tends to be the humans who put a spanner in the works. God put us here to be stewards and somehow along the way we lost the plot. Is it because of our arrogance, because we think we know better? This past year has shown us how much we are not in control of everything. Yet those who have coped the best are those who have found that balance within themselves. And that balance is not about shutting ourselves away but in reaching out to others. The planets in the sky achieve their balance by their relationship to the sun and to one another, we maintain our balance by our relationship to God and reaching out to each other.

Our journey through life is not a lone journey, it is a journey we take with the help and support of others and in turn our help and support to those around us. When we cut ourselves off we lose our way, because the way ahead is unknown and the only way to face it is together. We are at the opening of a New Year and we don't know what is ahead, we go there safe in the knowledge that we are not alone.

Kingsley

Sun 3 Jan

Subject: The Second Sunday of Christmas.

Dear Friends

John 1. 1-18. This is the greatest mystery of the Christian faith, and when I say mystery it is not hidden but in plain sight, it is just that it too wonderful to ever fully grasp. Jesus who is the Word of God, the Son of God, very God himself, entered the world where we live and breathe. Not a remote God but a God who we can know because we can know the Son, a God who wants to be called Father. And yet there is still pain and suffering in this world and so many unanswered questions, and perhaps this is part of the reason we find the mystery so hard to grasp.

On April 5th last year this email was no longer just to keep in touch, it became a daily email and our journey began. I freely admitted then that I did not have the answer and I still don't because no matter what some people say no one has the answer. But together we have explored the question and continue to do so.

God became a human being and lived as we live and his life was not easy and it was cut short, so we know he suffers with us. What we can't understand is why an all-powerful God allows suffering in the first place. I am not a theologian despite having a B.D. but a simple human being living in the world and not in a university. So together we still struggle with the question and in the end we have to simply trust he has his reasons. Put your hand in his hand and he will lead you through.

Kingsley

Mon 4 Jan

Subject: Week 41

Dear Friends

I have noticed that many people are more concerned and fearful. Christmas has come and gone, the New Year has started without being able to celebrate, and on our journey we face a long uphill climb. We still have a long way to go but at least we are on this journey together. Even now more and more people are joining our growing band and I am greatly encouraged by some of the responses I have had. When Mike, Sue and I walked the Pembrokeshire Coastal Path there were days when the wind and the driving rain made it hard going but we kept each other's spirits up and we eventually completed the 187 miles. The journey we are on now is not by choice, nor can we stop half way, it is a journey we are forced to finish and we can only encourage each other.

Continue to put one hand into the hand of God and the other into the people round you, walk confidently into the future, take today for what it brings and step by step we will get through.

Kingsley

Part 9
Dark Days

Tue 5 Jan

Dear Friends

All areas of England have now entered tier 4 as well, the numbers of those affected and the numbers of deaths are rising. Many churches have temporarily closed again and only provide online services. I will continue to hold services in St Mary's at 11.00 am every Sunday for those who still wish to come for the spiritual and mental welfare of those who need it, for the fellowship of meeting up while being very cautious. My only online presence is by this daily email, the responses to which I find really quite humbling. This is a hard stretch we face but it is only for a while.

Tomorrow is the celebration of the Epiphany when the magi visit Jesus, so perhaps today they are in Jerusalem. If only they had not gone to Jerusalem and met with Herod and set in motion a great evil. How many 'if only's' have there been throughout history. Even innocent and well intentioned actions have far reaching consequences. We must always remember that we are not in isolation and what we do does affect those around us. We can only try to do our best, do everything from a good heart, be a positive influence on those around us. Do not look for trouble, do not spread malicious gossip. Give freely, encourage one another, spread hope and joy.

The peace of God, which passes all understanding, keep your hearts and minds in the knowledge and love of God, and of his Son, Jesus Christ our Lord.

Kingsley

Wed 6 Jan

Subject: Epiphany

Dear Friends

I am sorry if I spoil your illusion of the stable scene with Mary and Joseph and the baby, the animals, the shepherds and the wise men all together. In Matthew the magi come to the house and only see Mary and Jesus, presumably Joseph is out working earning money to pay for the house where they were now living. We do tend to forget that these were real people who had to live day by day, they had to eat, they weren't tended on by angels all the time. And yet, wise men from the East had seen the star and had come to see this wonder, God on earth, and to bring gifts of gold, frankincense and myrrh, all of which had significance. The Christmas story is a mix of real life events and heavenly happenings and reminds us that there is far more going on than the world we can see, heaven does not intrude into our world but is a natural part of the greater reality we are not always aware of. The coming of the wise men heralds the revelation that is not just for the Jews but for everyone.

The word Epiphany has come to have an extra meaning, a moment of sudden and great revelation or realization. None of us are ever alone, we simply need to open our spiritual eyes and realise we are in God's presence and even if the worst happens in this world we are in his kingdom already.

Kingsley

Thu 7 Jan

Dear Friends

We still haven't had snow where I live, this morning is bright and sunny and a heavy frost covers everything, the branches of the leafless trees and hedges, the blades of grass on the lawn, the roofs of the few houses I can see, the distant fields across the valley. There is a stillness in the air. It is as if the world is waiting, and we are waiting too. We are waiting for the spring, we are waiting for a lessening of restrictions, we are waiting for better days. But we are not sitting around waiting, we are still getting on with life, but we are still waiting. I am not a patient person and I hate waiting, fortunately I am keeping busy. I am so glad the churches have not been forced to close this time and I am preparing for Sunday, I have a funeral today which I always find sad and I feel for the family, there are emails I need to respond to with church issues including the ones no longer used, wedding returns to fill in even though there have been none, occasional zoom meetings (yawn). The only time I am at peace with waiting is when I sit here and wait for inspiration, I need to be still at times despite myself. And I look forward to each new day, something new around the corner, maybe a chance meeting, perhaps today God will tell me what he expects, the wonderful emails I get back from this.

Have a good day.

Kingsley

Fri 8 Jan

Dear Friends

We get out of life what we put into it and I often wonder if our outlook in some way determines what happens to us. Being an over the top optimist myself I find good things always happen and if I was to believe in luck I would consider myself a very lucky person (don't ask me for next week's lottery numbers it isn't that sort of luck). And I wonder do pessimists create their own bad things or bad luck? Every morning I expect the day to be a good day and I find there is always something good in the worst of days. This isn't to say tragedy hasn't touched me or I haven't had major set-backs, just that there is always light at the end of every tunnel. In a way I suppose it is like when you are walking in the countryside, do you see the litter people throw out of their cars along the verges (I wonder what their houses are like), or do you see the new spring flowers beginning to show themselves, the green haze on trees where the buds are ready to burst forth with new leaves, do you hear the birds twittering in the bushes.

We do not live in a perfect world, God only pronounced everything good, and there are plenty of evil, greedy, selfish people about. But the good people need to make their presence felt in this world and overall the world will be a better place. And I am reminded of a quote that Ros has at the end of her emails, 'Our lives begin to end the day we become silent about things that matter.' from Martin Luther King Jnr. We will make a difference today.

Kingsley

Sat 9 Jan

Dear Friends

Time is still an enigma to me. In my book I have called the period between Easter and the end of April The Long Month, at the time I felt it would never end, time had really slowed down. And now we are well into 2021. I have appreciated this opportunity every day just to sit and be quiet and reflect, it has stopped time running away, I have been able to concentrate on each day as it came. This year has completely disrupted my conception of time, if someone asks about an event and how many years ago it was I have no idea. It seemed only a few days ago that Jesus was a baby and tomorrow he is getting baptised as an adult by John in the Jordan!

Time is the most precious gift we have, and when we give our time to someone it is worth more than any money. Once time is spent we cannot get it back and it so easy to waste it. There are things we put off until tomorrow and an opportunity is missed. Use today wisely.

Kingsley

Sun 10 Jan

Subject: The Baptism of Christ

Dear Friends

Mark 1. 4-11. Mark launches straight into John in fulfilment of Isaiah's prophecy preparing the way for the Lord by preaching and baptising in the desert. Jesus comes to him and is baptised at which point heaven is torn open, the Spirit descends on him as a dove and voice of the Father is heard pronouncing Jesus as his Son. This is a no nonsense statement of things as they happened. In later years the church was to make heavy weather of the Trinity, the books that have been written, the arguments, even a split between the Roman Church and the Orthodox Church. And why has the church decided to celebrate Jesus' baptism now? Straight after this Jesus goes off into the wilderness himself and yet we don't observe Lent until the end of February this year, we are still in Epiphany. Ah, but I am only a simple country Vicar and I don't expect to understand the thinking behind these things. I am also quite happy to accept Jesus being baptised by John and the Trinity being made plain for all to see.

It is alright to wonder, to question, even to doubt. But in the end God will do whatever God does and it all comes down to simple trust. We all feel so powerless at the moment, even afraid, we are children who do not understand, all we can do is trust. Put our hand into the hand of the Father and walk with faith into this new day.

Kingsley

Mon 11 Jan

Subject: Week 42

Dear Friends

I have often wondered what the point of envy is. To have what another person has you would have to be the other person and that means having their problems as well as their advantages, no one has a perfect life and we can only ever see part of anything. Money and possessions don't bring happiness, power brings responsibility, health and fitness requires hard work, celebrity means you are watched the whole time. What might look good on the outside might just be show. To have contentment is an important part of finding happiness, but this doesn't stop us having dreams and aspirations rather we know that we have to put in effort to achieve them. This pandemic has put much of our lives on hold but it has also given us the opportunity to think through what we really want and who we really are. This past year has only been a waste if you have done nothing with it. And if you have spent the time simply looking inward you have achieved nothing. It has often been said that we are in this together and when we forget this we have lost the plot, so much of who we are is our relationships with those around us even now.

Be the best person God wants you to be.

Kingsley

Tue 12 Jan

Dear Friends

With the numbers of COVID-19 cases still rising the rules are being enforced more stringently and there is a possibility that churches will be forced to close. We knew this was going to be a tough part of our journey but it is a journey and not a fixed place and this will pass. The vaccine is being given, the better weather is ahead, the days are lengthening. The human spirit is stronger that we often give ourselves credit for and we will win through. This is the hour of the wolf, when our fears are greatest, the night is dragging on and dawn seems never to be coming. But the earth rolls on without stopping and in time it will turn us to face the sun. This is a time of waiting which always seems longest but all time passes. Now is the time to encourage each other, to be there for one another, to give hope. It will soon be dawn.

Kingsley

Wed 13 Jan

Dear Friends

There seem to be a lot of people out walking these days, there are so many benefits in that. Not only is it good exercise, a chance to get out into the fresh air, but it also means you can meet people at a safe distance and have a chat. I feel for the people who live in places where they can't get out that easily. Computers and the internet are wonderful things, whenever I wake my computer up it greets me with a spectacular picture of somewhere in the world, but it is only a picture and it doesn't fill my whole vision, not like the world outside. So much of what we have had to do recently is on a screen but it is not the same as being there and meeting in person. I hope this isn't the way things will go in the future, I hope when we can travel and meet up in person we won't find it too convenient to continue doing things online. Even these emails will become unnecessary in time.

My big fear is that when this is over so much of what the church does will be online with the excuse that it reaches so many more people. Perhaps I am a dinosaur, perhaps I am mistaken if I think watching services comfortably in your own home lacks commitment, perhaps I am out of touch. I was told many years ago by a previous Archdeacon when I said I like to spend part of my week visiting people that those days have gone. When the restrictions have lifted I will continue to do my own thing even if it is out of step with everyone else. There are 15 churches I have gentle oversight of, I would like to come and visit, have a cup of coffee and a chat (not all at once). I will leave my computer at home and let it go to sleep.

Until we meet in person.

Kingsley

Thu 14 Jan

Dear Friends

We were warned that this second wave would be worse than the first and part of the reason is because it is winter. During the easing of the lockdown last summer I suppose we dared to hope the worst was over, we had a brief time when things were easy. But back through history winter has always been a tough time, the first Mesolithic settlers weren't sure they would even survive. But people are very resilient. We will get through this second wave and I still propose to have the service in the Cathedral after Easter to mark a year of these emails which have become a pilgrimage.

The days are perceptibly longer now, more noticeably on dry days. There is a lot of activity with the birds, I don't know when they actually build their nests but they are making a lot of noise in the hedgerows and the trees. The lawns are looking very long but it is too wet and too early to start mowing. Spring is gearing up to burst forth again. Nature all around us is getting on with life. Surely we can wait a little longer and in time the worst will pass and restrictions will be eased again. In the meantime don't forget to live today and appreciate what it holds.

Kingsley

Fri 15 Jan

Dear Friends

The latest from the Church in Wales yesterday is that in law we are not required to close churches and the Bench of Bishops are strongly advising that we find alternative ways rather than services in Church. By now you know my views on the matter, I will still be holding services in St Mary's every Sunday at 11.00 am but if anyone is concerned about attending there is no requirement for you to do so it is a personal choice. If that means I am the only one there then I will still be there and I will ring the bell.

Despite everything I still have my well of joy, I don't know where it comes from or why, nor can I stop it. I cannot help being optimistic and hopeful. Yes I know this is a worse wave than the first and more people are dying every day and I feel sad for them because they are not statistics but people with loved ones and each death affects so many around them, and I pray constantly that God will hold them in his hands. I know that many face uncertain futures, many businesses are struggling and some closing. I know that this is worse for children, their education and their futures. And yet ...

We will get through this, we will get on with our lives. The world still turns, time passes. We will greet each other with a cwtch, we will share a cup of tea and piece of cake, we will sing.

Joy to you today.

Kingsley

Sat 16 Jan

Dear Friends

Is it too soon to make plans? Is it too early to hope? The answer to these very much depends on where you are, the level of infections and the number of people being vaccinated. The next couple of weeks will surely give us a better idea of where we are, but can we begin to plan now? As you know I have arranged a Pilgrim Service with the Dean of the Cathedral for Saturday 10th April at 3.00 pm already and I am determined this will go ahead. Spring will be in full force by then and the hour will have changed. After that I will submit my emails again to the publisher for volume 2 and hope they are interested. So I already have plans. But we are not thinking about a holiday yet because there are still too many unknowns, and if we do go on holiday it will not be far.

It is never too early to hope, even in the saddest times there are reasons for that. Hope pushes us through the darkest hours and hope will see us through the next few weeks. The night is far gone, the day is at hand.

Kingsley

Sun 17 Jan

Subject: The Second Sunday of Epiphany

Dear Friends

John 1. 43-51. Jesus finds Philip and asks him to follow
him. Philip finds Nathanael and tells him about Jesus.
Nathanael is sceptical because Jesus is from Nazareth
until Jesus tells him he saw him under the fig tree, he
then declares Jesus to be the Son of God. This doesn't
sound like much to persuade someone, there must have
been something about Jesus that is not conveyed in the
passage that was compelling. Philip didn't need to
persuade Nathanael, only invite him to come, likewise it
is not up to us to persuade someone about faith in Jesus,
just point them in the right direction. Faith isn't about
clever arguments or reasoned theology or long sermons,
it is about giving someone the opportunity to meet with
Jesus. How do we do this? Simply be ourselves and let
the good news shine through us. It is how we live our
lives and the genuineness of our faith that will touch
others, it is not in our power to change a person's heart
or reach out to their soul. This is one of the reasons I
hope the church doesn't decide to do everything online
after the pandemic, it is far too impersonal, it is only
words. After all God didn't just sit in heaven and tell us
what to do, he entered the world and lived among us.
The internet is only a stop gap, the real work will be
done when we can meet and share on a personal level.
We will meet again and there will be such joy in that.

Kingsley

Mon 18 Jan

Subject: Week 43

Dear Friends

It was good to see so many in St Mary's yesterday, we are always careful and abide by the rules and it is good that we can still meet for worship. The number of COVID-19 cases is slowly easing and I know of people who are getting the vaccine today in Meddygfa Taf (Whitland surgery for those in foreign parts!). Perhaps at last we are over the worst.

We are all weary of this long journey and there is still a way to go but now at last we can see our destination in the distance. We have helped each other through this and we need to continue a while longer and let us not forget each other when times are easier, nor must we forget our local shops and the people who serve in them but continue to support them, and let us always remember all those who have gone out of their way to help. In time those who have lost loved ones during this difficult time will be able to mourn properly. Any celebrations we will have will always be tinged with sadness. But we will know we have got through this because we have been there for one another. One day soon we will all find our voices again and sing.

Kingsley

Tue 19 Jan

Dear Friends

As you go through life you pick up all sorts of pieces of information and you don't always remember where from. Just how much information can a brain hold? A bad memory is often down to our inability to find that dusty old memory that has been filed away, or too many similar things getting in the way, or simply lack of concentration at the time. Sometimes in the stillness memories pop into our conscious thought, sad memories, happy memories, decisions we made once and we wonder if we would make the same decision if we knew then what we do now. All our past experiences and the decisions we made, even our mistakes, have brought us to this point and we ask is this where we are where we want to be? My answer is yes, and that gives me such peace.

There are things we have no control over, such as the present pandemic, and we simply have to live through them. I am not a patient person but by being impatient is not going to affect the outcome so I learn to be still. I have been still for some time before typing away today, now is your chance to be still for a while.

Kingsley

Wed 20 Jan

Dear Friends

Two things that this pandemic is not. This is not one of the last plagues before the end of the world, there have been other pandemics throughout history and the world didn't end then nor will it now. This is not a judgement on the world or the church or anything else, the vulnerable have been worst hit not the people in power or the rich and famous. If anyone wants to disagree or argue with me then do so in two years time when this has become history. Don't be led astray by scare stories. It has given us an opportunity to reassess our lives and our faith, it has driven on technological advancements and medical science, it has changed the world and as with everything both good and bad will come as a result. The world goes on, life goes on.

The vaccine is being administered, infection rates are dropping, we have turned another corner and the road may still be rough but the end is in sight. Never despair, never give up hope, it will soon be dawn.

Kingsley

Thu 21 Jan

Dear Friends

In the Lord of the Rings as Frodo and Sam approach Mount Doom the weight of the ring drags Frodo down so much he can hardly put one foot in front of the other, Sam decides to carry him expecting to have the weight of the ring as well, but Frodo has lost so much weight he is light to carry and the weight of the ring is not a physical weight so Sam can easily carry him. Through difficult times perhaps we are required to carry someone else only to find it is easier than we thought because their burden is still their own and we are just there to help them through the dark patch. Many are going through darkness at the moment and even if we can do no more that hold the light we are helping. Be light for those in darkness, be hope for those who despair, be company for the lonely, be happiness and joy for the sad. Just be there.

Kingsley

Fri 22 Jan

Dear Friends

In these times of uncertainty and change it is comforting to know that there are some things that do not change and are certain. Day always follows night, Spring always follows Winter, a new moon always follows a waning moon, tides rise and fall, storms come and go, the sun is in the sky even when there are clouds and the wind will eventually blow the clouds away. The earth turns and the cosmic dance goes on. This may be the darkest stretch of our journey but there are still moments of joy, there are still surprises.

Yesterday I was in Llanfrynach Church for a funeral, and even for such a sad time there are moments when you can see beyond the darkness. I have been there before, some years ago for a harvest, but I had never before walked right up to the altar rail. It was like stepping through a door, all of a sudden I knew I was in a powerful presence, so very different to the presence of the angel in St Mary's. I cannot explain fully what it was and certainly not why it was there, except that it was a reminder that we are never alone, there is a reality beyond that which we can see. And this is something else that does not change, God and heaven and the spiritual realm are all around us and there is nothing humanity can do to affect this. Sometimes the thin veil is lifted for a moment and the light shines through.

Kingsley

Sat 23 Jan

Dear Friends

A heavy frost, a bright blue sky, the sun blazing away. This is the sort of winters day I love. Yet there is a sort of sadness in the air. I hear of more people who have had the first jab every day, the infection rate is falling, but there is no indication of what restrictions are going to be lifted or when. People are tired. And so it is with the last and hardest stretch of a journey, the stretch that seems to be never ending. If we look back we can see just how far we have come so perhaps it is worth pausing for a moment to reflect on what we have accomplished. Despite the restrictions perhaps there are people we have got to know better, perhaps made new contacts. Perhaps we have learned new technologies (though I still couldn't start a zoom meeting) or just become more comfortable with the technologies we know (I have found a way of putting in everyone's email address in one go!). Perhaps we have discovered the joys of walking and got to experience so much more of the nature about us. Perhaps we have found ourselves at a deeper level, (though no one has yet discovered my deeper level). We have not sat still. If future generations think this is a year when everything stopped they will be wrong, this is a year we have faced a challenge and we have got on with our lives.

Take courage, the journey will end, step out again today and live. Today is another day.

Kingsley

Sun 24 Jan

Subject: The Third Sunday of Epiphany

Dear Friends

John 2. 1-11. This is a fascinating event for many reasons. Jesus' mother goes to a wedding, no mention of his father so his mother was a widow now, and Jesus and his disciples are invited. You can imagine that Jesus was told to bring his friends and we have no idea how many disciples he had by now, no wonder they ran out of wine! When his mother mentions to him that they have run out of wine Jesus says it isn't his problem, he must be aware that his mother has told him for a reason because she knows what he is capable of. Then Mary puts Jesus on the spot by telling the caterers to do what he tells them. So he turns a huge amount of water into wine and only the stewards and some of his disciples know about this miracle, it is not an important miracle to prove a point and it is not instigated by Jesus, and how can providing more wine for party goers be a good thing? This shows a lot of humanity, it is simply a practical miracle. Not everything God does has to be impressive or startling or change someone's life. We see so many miracles in the natural world all the time that go unnoticed anyway. The world is full of endless wonder and we take so much for granted. See the magic in the every-day today, join the party that is all around.

Kingsley

Mon 25 Jan

Subject: Week 44

Dear Friends

We had a variety of weather yesterday. It began with such a heavy frost and the rain the night before had turned to ice, the gateway to St Mary's was like a bobsleigh track. There was freezing mist that made things worse. Later as it began to thaw it rained a little, then it hailed. Then I went up to Cyffig where there was snow on the ground and it hadn't cleared off the lane. And as I was coming back down the hill into Whitland there was a glorious rainbow as the sun shone on the drizzle. And the rainbow in the sky is a promise from God not to wipe us out with a flood, it is a reminder that the sun will come after the rain.

Today is dedicated to the conversion of Paul, a man of hate who was brought up short by being blinded on his way to Damascus in order that he might see. A man who had to reassess his whole life and in three days when his sight was given back his life had completely been turned around.

At the moment we live in dark days but God has set a rainbow in the sky, our lives have been turned around, has this year been a Damascus experience and have we learned?

Kingsley

Tue 26 Jan

Dear Friends

Although the vaccine is being administered people are realising it is not a magic potion, all it does is stop you becoming seriously ill, you can still catch the virus and you can still spread it. The governments still cannot give any idea of what restrictions will be lifted and when because they simply do not know. We are being told not to plan holidays. So people are beginning to murmur that we can write off this year as well. Oh dear, it all seems like doom and gloom, and I promised never to be like that. So where is that silver lining?

I never wrote off last year so I am not going to write off this year. It is simply that we cannot do lots of things that we took for granted, we have to live simpler lives, and is this such a bad thing? I admit is hard for people who are stuck indoors and have no social contact, but this is where neighbours and communities are so invaluable. It is hard for the sick and the bereaved. Yet life is still going on and I am still finding most people

I talk to are cheerful, in many ways despite social distancing we have drawn closer together. There are many people I have got to know much better during this time because people are more willing to share and talk about their concerns. The weather may be miserable today, the sky may be overcast, but with so much cloud there has to be a lot of silver linings. Live today with what it has to offer, find peace and do not give up on hope.

Kingsley

Wed 27 Jan

Dear Friends

Today is Holocaust Memorial Day, it is a day when we acknowledge that there is such evil in some people that they want to destroy an entire race. It is also a testament to the Jewish race that they survived and thrived. If we do not learn from history then we will make the same mistakes, and we must never turn a blind eye to the plight of others. I wonder how history will judge this present generation, did we do enough to protect the vulnerable, are we doing enough to give our children a future?

We do not have the advantage of hindsight, we simply live through these days. One thing that history does teach is that periods like this do pass, that people will live through them and rebuild their lives and society afterwards, we will rejoice we will be normal again, we will sing. And as I keep reminding you, there is still today and every day holds its own promise, expect something good today and you will find it.

Kingsley

Thu 28 Jan

Dear Friends

I was in a Zoom meeting yesterday for the LMA Deans. One of the things the Bishop told us was not to fast during Lent because this was a stressful enough time for us anyway. And I was thinking, 'what stress?' I know I am a calm person but despite the difficult times we are in I don't find it stressful, should I be? This is the most difficult part of our journey, and at times it is one foot in front of another as the lockdown drags on, but it is simply something we have to get through and continue to live our lives. One of the hardest things of this is that we cannot mix with our own families and friends and it is not the same over the phone, and the worst thing of all is not being able to visit loved ones in hospital. We cannot change anything by worrying about it, we continue to do the best we can in the circumstances and get on with living, looking for the wonders of each day, seeing the spring flowers opening up and the leaf buds growing on the trees and listening to the birds in the trees. In this world sadness and joy go hand in hand, it is simply the way of things. So don't get despondent, open your eyes to the glory all around.

Kingsley

Fri 29 Jan

Dear Friends

This pandemic has changed everything, it has taken away so much of what we were used to, everyone is having to adapt. So many are facing loss without being able to mourn properly, children are losing out on the fun and ease of social interaction and parents are having to be teachers, so many business are struggling or failing, even the shops that are allowed to be open have had to adapt to ways of managing things, so many illnesses are not being checked and mental health is an enormous issue. And it drags on. There has never been anything like this so how can anyone be an expert.

I have been given a calm disposition and a well of joy that seems bottomless, so I do the only thing I can. I try to be a little voice of hope, a little spark of light. We each of us have our gifts and perhaps mine have been given for such a time as this. All I can do is encourage, remind you of the magic and the wonder of each day, and be here at the other end of the emails if you need an ear (or rather an eye), and I can pray. I can also spread the good news I hear of the tremendous good that is being done all the time by people in the community, there is always far more good things than bad in this world even, and especially, in dark times like these. We are in the final push of our journey and we will finish it.

Kingsley

Sat 30 Jan

Dear Friends

Yesterday in Wales any easing of restrictions were so slight it reminds us that we still have a long way to go. One thing I am grateful for is that the government didn't force the churches to close when we entered this latest lockdown back in December, it is a place for people to meet if they wish, it is a sign to the community that we are still here, and it does give some structure to my week and something to aim for. The rest of the week I am still never sure what day it is. Time has become so muddled that if I try to work out how many years ago something was, especially if it was only two or three years, I just can't work it out. This has gone on so long now the memory of the previous normal life is beginning to fade. Have I got stuck in a rut? With all the things we can't do have our worlds become small?

We have all been given an imagination, the ability to lift ourselves out of the confines of where we are, to expand our world even when we physically can't. And we have a spirit that is free and no amount of restrictions can tie us down. We have a heart that can love at any distance and can reach right around the world to people we know and have compassion for people we don't. We have our intellect, our ability to learn new things all the time and expand our horizon and our fount of knowledge. We have the tools to be free so let us use them.

Kingsley

Sun 31 Jan

Subject: The Fourth Sunday of Epiphany

Dear Friends

Mark 1: 21-28. Jesus was teaching in the synagogue and people were amazed at him because he had authority unlike the teachers of the law. Then when confronted by a man with a demon he told the demon to leave the man, and people were even more amazed at this authority too. Fine words, often heaps of them, and reasoned arguments are all very well but how often do we hear anyone preach with authority? I suppose we would know the answer if we actually heard it, but I find it difficult to trawl through my memory for one really outstanding sermon. Perhaps I am being unfair, or too critical, or have too short a memory.

All through this pandemic I have not heard one rousing speech, one authoritative voice. Are people too busy talking to listen to what God has to say? In the silence all I can hear is, 'If you fall I will catch you.'

Kingsley

Mon 1 Feb

Subject: Week 45

Dear Friends

Yesterday the Bishop held her Visitation via Zoom. I missed getting in a car with the Wardens and driving to a gathering in a large Church, I missed meeting up with friends I haven't seen for a while. With over 200 little faces spread over 7 screens, watching from my study, there was no togetherness, no atmosphere, I might just as well be watching the news. In short, I cannot get used to this and I will never feel comfortable with it.

Yesterday we had snow, not a lot and it is mostly gone today, just enough to make the roads rather slushy and make it difficult for some people to get to St Mary's. Still it was good to see those who did come.

This pandemic has done so much damage, all those who have died, all those who have lost loved ones, all those who have lost jobs, all those who are cut off, all those who suffer physically and mentally. This is week 45 since the beginning of the first lockdown and if we are not careful we will lose the art of social interaction. When this is over perhaps we should shut off our computers and get back out into the real world.

This evening in the Celtic year it is Imbolc, the beginning of spring, the promise of new life and fruitfulness. It is a time of possibilities, a time of reawakening. A time of renewed hope. Let the seed of joy grow in your hearts, let the real world begin again in us.

Kingsley

Tue 2 Feb

Dear Friends

This is where the church calendar really confuses me, the naming of Jesus was 1st Jan, now today we have his presentation in the temple or Candlemas, Luke 2: 21 says he was circumcised on the eighth day, and purification in Jewish law was seven days so I remain confused as to why Candlemas is today and not 1st Jan. Ah well, they must have had their reasons, so I won't say it is to Christianise a pagan festival.

At least the government is saying we will be able to enjoy summer, well I am going to enjoy the spring. From my window I can see the early signs of spring everywhere, the window where I have looked out and typed away every day and watched the changing seasons and have taken time to reflect. I have seen nature get on with life, the changing colours of the leaves, the coming and going of the wild flowers, the birds flying to and fro. I have seen people passing, walking along the Roman Road, in the summer in their light clothes and now all wrapped up in warm coats. I have seen the sun rise and fall and begin his journey again. I have seen the rains and the mists and on Sunday even snow, the grey skies and the blue. And soon the green haze on the trees will reveal the new leaves, the bright fresh green.

While the earth remains, seedtime and harvest, cold and heat, summer and winter, day and night, shall not cease. Gen 8. 22

Kingsley

Wed 3 Feb

Dear Friends

When I write about the weather it is only a local thing, I am aware that many of you are many miles away and that in Canada you are having snow storms and in Australia it is summer. Modern technology is a wonderful thing even though I am somewhat of a technophobe for its ability to keep the whole world in touch in an instant. For all that I hate Zoom it is a useful tool to keep things going, and the internet and phone systems have been vital at this time for people to keep in touch with each other. I still look forward to the day when I can drop in on someone and have a coffee or tea (a little milk and no sugar and please don't pile cakes on me). I am informed that you cannot bless the communion via the internet, but I thought that was obvious, any more than sharing a cup of tea can be done over the internet, the sharing of any meal is a very personal and intimate event and has to be done in person.

Nature doesn't do technology yet birds can fly thousands of miles and find the nest they made last year, the seasons are governed by the position of the sun, the tides by the moon, the rain clouds by the winds, and all the little wild animals know when to go about their business. We are surrounded by endless wonder and we do need to take our eyes off the screen. We need to come together as soon as we can because this is what it is to be human and not robots.

Part 10
New Hope

Kingsley

Thu 4 Feb

Dear Friends

A mother and two small children just walked past on the Roman Road, the older holding the reigns of the younger who couldn't have been walking long. Events in our very early life affect us well into adulthood and very often we don't even remember the events. The effects of this pandemic are going to be with us for a very long time and many of them unseen. Already the mental health of so many people has been affected, and the strain is beginning to tell on many others.

One of the big subjects of conversation at the moment is 'have you had your jab yet?' and 'any ill effects?'. People keep asking me if I have had the jab yet but I point out Vicars are not care workers, it isn't a medical necessity for us to visit, even if some people would argue it is on spiritual or mental health grounds, and we do not want to be seen as queue jumpers. I am content to wait my turn, there are people with greater need.

With the vaccine proving even better than expected there is more hope about that at some point we will return to normal.

We must continue to take one day at a time, deal with whatever is, be aware of the needs and concerns of others, and be prepared for the problems of the future. We continue to live in the present and look for the magic in each day, there is still so much more good than bad, so much to be thankful for.

Kingsley

Fri 5 Feb

Dear Friends

I must be on a different planet to everyone else, not only am I a self-confessed technophobe but if someone starts to ask me if I watched ... I tend to say no before they get as far as saying what it was because I don't watch television apart from the New Year's concert from Vienna and I did watch the Pembrokeshire Murders mini-series. Jo-an and I like remote holidays on Scottish islands away from it all because of the slower pace of life, my idea of extreme boredom is lying on a beach and doing nothing, and I am not a party animal. You already know I am not stressed or fearful, and I do not believe that although the church shot itself in the foot that this is the end of the church, it will come back because I have seen the dedication of the local people concerning their local church. Whatever people think of the church it is a presence, it is a structure that God can work through and we do not need to reinvent the wheel. The message I has the other day is still ringing in my ears, 'If you fall I will catch you.'

You may also like to know that The Queen appreciated the book and sends you all her best wishes.

Kingsley

Sat 6 Feb

Dear Friends

When these emails started it was by chance rather than plan, and although it now reaches so many people in so many countries it is still only a relatively small number. I am only one small voice of hope and I am sure there are many other small voices of hope scattered all over. We all encourage each other. And now as the latest peak has passed and the numbers of cases is slowly dropping and hopefully the number of death will follow there is a general feeling that we may return to some sort of normality, yet people know this may still be a long way off and are talking about months not weeks. Last summer I suppose we dared to hope the worst was over, this year we are far more cautious.

The world is all about cycles, the changing seasons, day and night, and for all the wonders of modern life we are still people living in the world, part of nature and our lives are affected by cycles all the time. We are not stuck in one place, and every hard or dark period will always be followed by an easier lighter time. Even death is not the end because of the promise of heaven. Today is another day and we will live today for the joys it holds, we have reasons for hope so let us smile.

Kingsley

Sun 7 Feb

Subject: Creation Sunday

Dear Friends

John 1. 1-14. God created through his Word, in Genesis when God said it came to be and in John's Gospel we read that this Word became flesh and dwelt among us and we know him as Jesus. Yet the world did not recognise him and his own did not receive him. Of all mysteries this is the deepest because all our unanswered questions arise out of this. When God created the world he saw that it was good, why not perfect? In the gap between good and perfect he has given us choice which we would not have had in a perfect world, he didn't want us to love him simply because we had no choice but because we wanted to. In that gap was always the possibility of rejection, which is why Jesus was rejected and executed, and this was always part of the plan so that the option of repentance and forgiveness is always open. The choice was not simply a once and for all choice, not for us humans anyway. Yet the choice people make to go their own way and reject God has led to so much evil. Do we blame God for giving us free will? Forgive me for being rather deep today, this is something I have always struggled with.

Always remember that God made the world and it was and is good. Look at the world about us and see there is far more good than bad, and above this there is always hope. Make good choices.

Kingsley

Mon 8 Feb

Subject: Week 46

Dear Friends

The lockdown drags on and all we look forward to at the moment is the slow lifting of restrictions. This part of the journey is a hard slog and we can't really plan for a future we don't know what it will be. I am still hoping for the Pilgrim Service in the Cathedral but it would be nice to plan some sort of celebration, yet we don't know what we will be allowed by then. We need some magic, we need something really exciting to look forward to. We probably all have things we would like to do, things we took for granted before the pandemic, and just to be able to do these simple things again will be good. When we can do the simple things we used to do such as getting together with family and friends, when we can greet each other with a cwtch, when we can sing, we will appreciate these things all the more and it will be in these simple things that we will find joy. Yet it is still worth expecting joy today, looking for the magic in the present. We have some measure of hope with the vaccine being administered to more and more people and the passing of the latest peak. So let us hope and dream, let us be glad for today, let us live and step forward into the future.

Kingsley

Tue 9 Feb

Dear Friends

When C.S. Lewis wrote 'The Lion, the Witch and the Wardrobe' for Lucy he realised she was already getting too old for fairy stories but hoped one day she would be old enough for them again. Is it wrong to believe in things we cannot see, things science tells us do not exist? Is it wrong to believe that many legends and myths have some basis in truth? All faiths are based on beliefs that cannot be proved and the universe about us is so vast and complex and full of wonder no one can possibly know everything and there are experiences that rational people have had that there is no scientific answer to. Science after all is only the study of things that can be repeated and examined and there is so much that cannot be tested in this way.

In these day when we are unable to do so much at least we are fee in our minds, we can dream and no one can stop us, we can believe in our hearts and no one can take that away, we are not bound by social distance in our spirit. Being a dreamer, believing in five impossible things before breakfast, this has kept me not only sane but full of joy and hope so it can't be wrong. Unless I am actually mad and no one has the heart to tell me.

Kingsley

Wed 10 Feb

Dear Friends

Something I am hearing quite a lot now is COVID fatigue, this has gone on so long now and even though the vaccine is rolling out and the numbers of cases are falling there is no clear way out of this and more and more people are weary. On a long pilgrimage even when you know you are near your destination you become weary, the last stretch seemingly goes on for ever because now you are keen to set down your burden and relax yet there is still a distance to go. We have come so far, we have been through dark times, things are looking more promising and we are keen to get on with our lives again. But we still do not know what the future is going to be like and we cannot make too many plans, so perhaps there is a certain amount of trepidation too. The future is always uncharted territory anyway but since we are living through an experience we could not be prepared for the future is so much more of an unknown.

Since I have somehow fallen into the role of cheerer up you will either be annoyed or encouraged to know I don't have COVID fatigue, nor does the future bother me. I make things up as I go along anyway, even when faced with a difficult meeting I never plan what I am going to say. The future unrolls as it will, as it always has done, we have got this far through so many futures at the time and we will meet the futures that are yet to be. We are all more capable than sometimes we give ourselves credit for and we will cope with whatever comes. Do not give in to fatigue, do not be downhearted, step with confidence into today and tomorrow and all the tomorrows, God is your guide and he trusts you too.

Kingsley

Thu 11 Feb

Dear Friends

Recently a Lawyer in Texas made a court appearance on Zoom as a cat, I must try and find out how to do that so that for my next Zoom meeting I can appear as something, it would be good if everyone did that it would make Zoom meetings a bit more fun. The trouble now is for my next Zoom meeting I will be trying to imagine what everyone would choose to be and I won't take it seriously. Sometimes we need a bit of light-hearted relief, this doesn't distract us from what is serious, people are still suffering and dying, people are still facing an uncertain future, but we just cannot be too intense all the time. I must admit I have an odd sense of humour, I don't find stand-up comedians funny, while natural humour or unintentional humour gets me laughing, often in the wrong place. I wonder what is the point of humour and laughter, why do we have it? If we are in the image of God then he must have a sense of humour too. After all, I am sure some of the things Jesus said were meant to be amusing and I expect his hearers laughed. Oh dear, I have probably just upset the straight laced people who wear black to go to church and sit there with long faces.

But read Ecclesiastes 3.4 a time to weep and a time to laugh, a time to mourn and a time to dance,. And such is life that sometimes these times can come on top of each other.

Kingsley

Fri 12 Feb

Dear Friends

When I moved house recently I took the opportunity to throw a lot of stuff out, yet I still had one of the bedrooms piled high with bags and boxes which I have been slowly going through and I am still getting rid of things. Since the beginning of the first lockdown I have taken the opportunity to go through some of my mental and spiritual baggage and some of my preconceived ideas. I have had a good re-think about many things including, as you have probably noticed, church traditions especially ones I blame the Romans for! Faith of any sort is not complicated, it is really quite simple and it is very personal, I don't expect you to believe what I believe. Faith is simply a relationship with God, understanding where we fit into this world. When I moved house and when I still go through the clutter in the bedroom I can physically see the things that I have accumulated, a spiritual spring clean is not so easy because we don't always know where our ideas come from. As the days lengthen and get brighter we can see the dust and sweep it out. We need to let the light into our souls so we can sweep the dust out of there too. With Lent fast approaching now is a good time to have a spiritual spring clean.

Kingsley

Sat 13 Feb

Dear Friends

With snow lying round about it looks like a Christmas card today. We have been told two hopeful things, one is that it is hoped we will have the same freedoms this summer as we did last summer, the other that by next winter we will be able to live with the virus as we live with flu. From about Easter many things will be allowed to open again so I am still aiming for the Pilgrim Service in the Cathedral on 10th April. In addition the Bank of England says the country is like a coiled spring ready to bounce back. Wales has reached its target offering the vaccine for over 70's two days early so the over 65's are next. And for all of you who have asked for a second book I have high hopes for that too.

The other interesting piece of news is that the stones of Stone Henge were not only taken from the Preseli Mountains but they formed a stone circle there too and were later moved, but I already knew that, and not only from Waun Mawn.

I wonder what news today will bring.

Kingsley

Sun 14 Feb

Subject: Transfiguration Sunday

Dear Friends

Mark 9. 2-9. Jesus takes Peter, James and John up a mountain, there he is transfigured before them and he meets Moses and Elijah. For a moment they see beyond the physical world to who Jesus really was and that death is not the end, there is a greater reality beyond. When we talk about ourselves having a dual nature, of being physical and spiritual, of there only being a veil between us and the otherworld, have we fully grasped what that means? No, because we are bound to this physical world as we should be and a glimpse is all we get if we get that at all, sometimes in a thin place we have a feeling or an impression and no more. Because if we really realised what is beyond we would be so caught up in heavenly things we would forget to live in the present. Peter James and John were given this insight as a promise to keep them through the hard times that were to come, they continued to live their lives and even to doubt at times, but they had a mission ahead of them.

There are times that we need to be reminded of who we are, that we are much more than the physical beings living our lives in this world, to raise us out of despondency and despair, but not so much that we forget we still have a life in this world and while we live we have a purpose, a mission to show the kingdom through our actions and words. We are lights in a dark place, so let us live fully in this world knowing we are more than what we are without being so heavenly minded that we are no earthly good. This is still a good and beautiful world and we are to have joy in the present.

Kingsley

Mon 15 Feb

Subject: Week 47

Dear Friends

Time is creeping by and one day we will be able to look back at this period in our lives. Sometimes I wonder how we will remember it and I will be glad I kept a record, but that is not yet. Yesterday was also St Valentine's Day and it is hard to think that only a year ago Jo-an and I went out for a meal and as it turned out that was the last time we did. Only a year but it seems so much longer, and apart from Sundays because I am in church I still get confused as to what day of the week it is. Life changes all the time, normally the changes happen gradually and we don't notice until we look back, this change was forced on us suddenly and I don't suppose anyone has really come to terms with it because so much is against our instincts. We cannot meet together or pop in to see friends, we have to keep our distance and often step aside when passing someone we know on the road, we cannot sing. One day we will be able to meet together and pop in to see friends, one day the tape will be removed, one day we will even be able to dispense with the masks and one day we will sing again. When we can we must not be afraid to do so. As it is the days are getting longer, spring is in the air and there is more hope now than perhaps a month ago. Enjoy what today brings for every day is a gift.

Kingsley

Tue 16 Feb

Subject: Shrove Tuesday

Dear Friends

Today is Shrove Tuesday when traditionally everything you would give up for Lent would be put in a pan and cooked together to use it up. I must say I don't fancy a pancake made of cake, chocolate and alcohol or whatever else people tend to give up these days. For myself I can never think of what to give up, rather I try to do something constructive, perhaps study more or reflect more which is exactly what I have been doing since last Lent anyway. So how will I mark Lent this year? Perhaps my reflections will be a bit deeper? We will have to see what develops. I find there is much more hope in people these days, so it is not a time to wear sackcloth and look miserable, rather this Lent let us look for the positive.

In the early church those wishing to be baptised would be taken to a place where they could be taught what it meant to be a follower of Jesus, this was a new faith after all and often had to be practiced in secret. The rest of the church would pray for those under instruction and surely it would be a joyous time for so many more were being added to their number. This would have been a hopeful time for the growing church. Our prayer at this time should be that since this is God's Church (Not Catholic, Orthodox, Anglican, Baptist, Presbyterian, Methodist, etc.,) he can breathe life into the Church again, and "here we are, use us."

Kingsley

Part 11
Lent

Subject: Ash Wednesday

Dear Friends

With all the hopeful signs for an end to the lockdown, with the falling number of infections and deaths, we are still here in the middle of it. I have read a new thing, it is called 'compassion fatigue' where human beings protect themselves by going numb because of the number of deaths, and we are told it is OK to be not OK. Every day I look up the daily deaths numbers in the UK and in Wales and say a silent prayer and although there are fewer now than there were every death is a sadness, every death is a person with family and friends and I try not to be numb to this while at the same time looking for the positive to say every day. On this Ash Wednesday and throughout Lent spare a prayer for all who suffer, this is far better than giving up something for Lent.

Meanwhile life does go on, we may be missing the little things we took for granted but we can still find things that give us joy. There is still the telephone to keep in touch with loved ones, there are still the chance meetings when we go out for a walk, there is also the opportunity to catch up with things we were too busy to do before. There is spring all around us, primroses, daffodils, snowdrops and people have even seen crocuses, some of the sparrows on the bird feeder are looking very fat and not being an expert I was wondering if they were ready to lay eggs. The days are lengthening too. In your keenness to look to the future do not forget to look at the wonders of the world about you each day.

Have a good day.

Kingsley

Thu 18 Feb

Dear Friends

When I began these emails I never promised answers, in all my dealings with people I have found that what may be an answer for someone is no answer for someone else, and I have to admit I am one of those awkward people who are irritated by people who always have an answer and know everything. One of the best pieces of advice I had when I was in Theological College was from a retired priest who said sometimes it is best just to sit with someone and say nothing, he had sat and said nothing for an hour with a woman once whose son had committed suicide, he left feeling he had failed her, a year later he bumped into her in Tesco's and she thanked him for how he helped her. People need to find their own answers. Have you noticed Jesus never gave any answers, he only asked other questions.

We will never have an answer to why this pandemic happened and why so many people died. What will always rankle with me is that all of a sudden the church was not there, which is why I have kept St Mary's and Cyffig open now, and I hope in some small way these emails have been me sitting with you through all of this, and I really appreciate all of you sitting with me too. Together you and I will get through this, drawing strength from each other. Let us sit together today for a while, even if we say nothing.

God bless you all.

Kingsley

Fri 19 Feb

Dear Friends

It is alright to cry. I have known funerals when relatives have not cried either because it has been a happy release or they have gone to a better place, they do not cry because they do not want others to see them cry because of their strong faith. We are all going through bereavement at the moment, some people have lost loved ones and for them it is much worse but we have all lost a way of life. I know I have tried to be positive throughout and generally speaking I am, it is not an act, but I do mourn the things I have lost. We all have human hearts, this is a delicate thing, with it we fall in love and it is so fragile it can break. It is also alright to laugh, even at a funeral, and throughout this pandemic there have been occasions for joy and laughter. Life is not a drab monochrome, it has its ups and downs, and this world is still a place of endless wonder.

I wish you joy today.

Kingsley

Sat 20 Feb

Dear Friends

I must admit I am not a patient person, I don't like hanging about but would rather get on with things. At present we have no choice but to be patient, we know the end is coming but it is not yet and is still a way off. In many ways we had got used to things happening immediately and because of technology a lot of things still do. On our pilgrimage we can see the end in the distance but we still have a lot of travelling before we get there. So although we are tired, we are pushing on against fatigue, with every step we do get closer. The distant haven may not look as if it is getting nearer but every day it is. If we were physically together on this journey we could do so much more to bolster each other's spirits, we could sing a walking song. The hardest part of all this is our remoteness from one another, technology is a wonderful thing but it will never replace personal contact. And this is something we need to remember when this is over, online is no substitute for fellowship. So I look forward to meeting up with as many of you as possible, some of you are from such far flung places this may not happen, but all of us will be able to meet up with friends and family again, we will all be able share personally again, we will be able to cwtch and we will be able to sing. walk on, walk on with hope in your hearts and you'll never walk alone.

Kingsley

Sun 21 Feb

Subject: First Sunday of Lent

Dear Friends

Mark 1. 9-15. Mark's account of Jesus in the desert for forty days is typically brief, only two verses, he was tempted by Satan, he was with the wild animals, and angels attended him. Matthew and Luke go into the details of the temptations, only Mark mentions the wild animals. So if you are wondering what wild animals and are thinking perhaps rabbits and badgers then it is worth knowing that there were lions and bears. Yet the danger was not from the lions and bears but from Satan and from his own thoughts. Later on, during his ministry, Jesus warned that evil does not come from outside but from within a person's own heart. We cannot blame our circumstances for how we are but how we deal with circumstances. We are all still going through a really difficult challenge so no one can feel any more hard done by than anyone else, it is how we have dealt with this pandemic and the lockdowns that show what we are truly made of.

And don't forget, angels attended him, Matthew also mentions this. We are not alone, even in our darkest days there is light and hope and joy if only we can see it. We should shut our minds to Satan, simply live with the lions and bears, and open our hearts to wonders we cannot see.

Kingsley

Mon 22 Feb

Subject: Week 48

Dear Friends

There is a strange mixture of feelings about. This present situation is really dragging on and people are fed up and weary, eager to get on with normal things again, while there is more hope about that the restrictions will lift in time, the vaccine is reaching more and more people and the death rate is falling yet every death is still a person with a family, and our leaders are beginning to make hopeful statements. And still we plod on day by day, and time is still passing.

I am still enjoying my little rambling away every day, I am still amazed that people are reading them and even asking when the second book will be available! This is still an interesting journey with many sights to be seen along the way, sometimes I wish I was more of an expert on flora and fauna so I could describe better the sights I see from my window with the changing seasons. Obviously the birds have not heard of the ban on singing because they are flat out at the moment. Spring is a time for new beginnings, for new life, when our spring eventually arrives let us make the most of it, let us live life to the full, let us give thanks and rejoice. This day will come.

Kingsley

Tue 23 Feb

Dear Friends

Although February is the shortest month of the year it still seems to drag at the best of times because although there are signs of spring everywhere winter still refuses to let go. And now is certainly not the best of times, and this pandemic is refusing to let go even with all the hopeful signs that it is easing. I consider myself very fortunate to have such a positive outlook that even February can't dampen me, but I am fully aware that this is not so for everyone. This is a hard time for many of you and you can't just snap out of it, this is still a hard slog and is wearing people down. Do not be afraid to admit you find it hard to cope and remember that although I can't physically come and see you I am here if you need me, this was the original point of these emails anyway nearly a year ago.

Hobgoblin nor foul fiend can daunt my spirit. If I could spread the well of joy I would. I can at least remind you again that day follows night, the sun is still there even when it is cloudy, God is still there even in the darkness of our spirits. We all need something magical now, some bright happening especially now as the end seems so far away. There is a treasure today, see if you can find it.

Kingsley

Wed 24 Feb

Dear Friends

I may not be a morning person but every day I wake up with an air of expectancy. Today is going to be a good day. I am going to learn something new, I may meet someone or hear from someone I haven't seen for a while, I am going to hear some news along the way. Every day is another step along the journey and rather than look back at what has gone I look to the hope we all have when restrictions are eased, and I enjoy the day that I live through now. I still view this as a pilgrimage and each day has something to teach us about ourselves, about others and about the world around us. Spring continues to advance and even on a drab day like today the birds are in full song. If it isn't raining too much I shall walk down to the town for the paper and one or two necessities this morning, a walk I always enjoy. With all the sadness, loss and darkness this world is still full of endless wonder, it is full of magic. Do not let the good things slip past unnoticed.

Kingsley

Thu 25 Feb

Dear Friends

I have always maintained this pandemic was not caused by God, it is not a judgement on anyone, it is a consequence of people messing with nature. We had hoped that the world would become a better place but it is no better or worse. Many people have taken the opportunity to reflect, to rethink, but we always fill our time with things and rarely have we been still enough to hear God. It feels like we have been on this pilgrimage without a map and without a compass but somehow we are being guided through it. Our faith has been tested and hopeful it will be stronger. We still have questions and the future is still uncertain. I never pretended to know the answer, and it is still my constant prayer that God will reveal something, what is more I believe he will but not yet. When Elijah hid in the mountain God was not in the wind, the earthquake or the fire but in the still small voice and what he said to Elijah in that small voice changed everything. This time when God speaks it will not be what we expect, for the old has gone, it has been wiped away, now is a time of rebirth. Easter is approaching, let us make it mean something special, let us prepare our hearts, let us recover joy and hope and face the new world with confidence.

Kingsley

Fri 26 Feb

Dear Friends

For almost a year we have been living with a sense of unreality, so much has changed that although we have learned to live with things as they are we still have not got used to it. It is as if we stepped through a door into a world that is like ours but is not ours. No wonder so many people feel unsettled. At the same time nature all around us is unaffected, the seasons have followed their usual course, the weather continues to be unpredictable, the spring flowers are emerging all over the place, the birds are busy doing what birds do at this time of year. The sun rises and sets, the moon goes through her cycle, the stars in the sky are the usual ones for this time of year. In a cosmic sense we are of no importance and the universe around us is unaffected by us. The only way we can have meaning at all is in God we are loved and important to his plan, whatever that is. This means all those who have died are important too and whatever happens so much we have to take on faith. Faith itself can be elusive and many things can make us doubt and question. This pandemic has thrown up so many questions and we cannot pretend we do not have them, our faith is tested and we cannot pretend it hasn't or fall back on stock Bible quotes to cover over the cracks. Yet this I know beyond a shadow of a doubt, when we fall he will catch us, when we doubt he is there, when he wipes the tears from our eyes he keeps them and treasures them.

Kingsley

Sat 27 Feb

Dear Friends

Our pilgrimage has also been a voyage of discovery. Because we do not know the future each step is a step into the unknown. We need to let the past go, it will not come again and we cannot rebuild what has gone. If we have been listening we have also been discovering a lot about ourselves. If we have not changed then we have truly wasted a year for whatever else this pandemic has been it has been an opportunity for us to explore ourselves and our outlook on life and indeed our beliefs. But it hasn't been about simply looking inward at ourselves rather how we care about all those around us. Many times in these emails, especially in the early ones, I have said we have been given a blank canvass on which to paint a new future particularly for the church.

Therefore make the most of today, look at the wonders around, realise how far we have come already and continue forward with confidence. We are not the people who were placed in lockdown nearly a year ago, time to stretch out as the new people we are now. The night is far gone, the dawn is approaching, time for us to live again, to hope and to dream and to plan.

Kingsley

Sun 28 Feb

Subject: The Second Sunday of Lent

Dear Friends

Mark 8. 31-38. Jesus predicts his death, Peter rebukes him and Jesus rebukes Peter saying, "Get behind me, Satan!", and goes on to tell the crowd the cost of being a disciple. Jesus never promised an easy life and sometimes he does expect so much from us, and it is tempting when we see others seemingly have everything. Yet nothing of any lasting value has ever been easy, true rewards take time and effort rather than the fleeting pleasures of the moment that do not last. In today's reading Peter had only just before said that he knew Jesus was the Christ, but he had misunderstood what that meant and still thought in worldly terms, how could the Christ be killed? God's plans are long term plans not for just the moment and from our perspective we find it hard to understand them. We must simply trust, hard though it is. The present may be difficult, the road rough, but God will see us through. The pandemic will end, the signs are already here, we are on the verge of a new beginning.

Kingsley

Mon 1 Mar

Subject: Week 49

Dear Friends

Happy St David's Day. "Lords, brothers and sisters, Be joyful, and keep your faith and your creed, and do the little things that you have seen me do and heard about. And as for me, I will walk the path that our fathers have trod before us."

Often people want to do the big things, to make a loud pronouncement, to be noticed and as Jesus said they have received their reward, the transient reward of fame in the moment. The reward of the little things, on the other hand, is eternal. Far more good is done quietly without show. It is a strange thing that with some people the more you do for them the more they take for granted while it is the little acts of kindness that almost pass unnoticed that are the most appreciated. I have always found that it is not the people who make a show of their good works that do the most good, but the people who quietly get on with helping others. From our perspective it may seem like God turns everything upside down but surely it is us who view things the wrong way. Fame is so fleeting and means nothing, it is who we are that endures.

Today in memory of St David, let us do the little things that make the world a far better place.

Kingsley

Tue 2 Mar

Dear Friends

In this corner of the world we are enjoying a spell of bright sunny weather, there are a lot of people walking along the Roman Road like they were during the first lockdown. We didn't know at that time this would go on so long, yet here we are almost a year later. Dare we hope that when the restrictions are lifted they won't have to be re-imposed? No one here has a crystal ball do they? We continue to live from day to day, we continue to have hope, we look for the magic in every day and find joy in the small things. It is worth beginning to plan for the future, I am working out a rota for Holy Week and Easter so I can get round all five of my immediate churches and I am still looking forward to the Pilgrim Service in the Cathedral on 10th of April. I am toying with planning a holiday but I don't intend to go far, after all Wales is such a beautiful country why go anywhere else? On our long pilgrimage the road now is a little smoother and the end is getting closer, let us take in the sights and sounds of today, let us smile and sing in our hearts, dawn is beginning to break.

Kingsley

Wed 3 Mar

Dear Friends

Yesterday I had my first vaccine jab, I walked down in the bright sunshine to Meddygfa Taf, waited a little, went in for the slight scratch of the Oxford one, and walked back up again. No ill effects at all, I am lucky like that. I feel like I passed a milestone. Sadly our spell of nice weather has abruptly come to an end as it is raining out now. Ah well, we can't expect sunshine all the time. Every day is different and it is always a mixture of good and bad, but always the good is far greater. Life is always a balance, we need to get on with our lives in the physical reality while taking care of our spiritual side too. We are whole beings, not one thing or the other but a complex mix of so many things. When we talk about our heart it is the vital organ that keeps blood flowing through our bodies to keep us alive, and it is also the centre of our emotions that make us human beings, a vital part of who we are and how we relate to all those around us. Look after yourselves today in all the complex aspects of who you are, and above all make the most of all that is good.

Kingsley

Thu 4 Mar

Dear Friends

Sometimes the timing of events seem planned and I wonder how different things could have been if things hadn't happened when they did. One example is the formation of this Local Ministry Area, I had originally turned down the post of LMA Dean saying it was impossible to form the proposed group with just two clergy and was eventually persuaded to accept on the promise a third cleric would be found (still waiting). Representatives of the fifteen churches had met and I managed to get at least one email from someone in each church. The inauguration service took place in February last year so I was officially LMA Dean but we still hadn't set up a council or appointed any officers and because of the lockdowns we still haven't. If none of the above had happened I would have just been responsible for my five churches and wouldn't have tried to keep in touch with the whole area. This has given me a purpose throughout this last year and continues to do so, this has kept me in touch with so many people. My world could have been so much smaller.

Events in life always have consequences, if your intentions in the beginning are good then surely what follows will be mostly good too. If your intentions in the beginning are mean and selfish then who knows what evil will follow. You reap what you sow, the wheel turns and what you put into life you generally get back. Sadly this doesn't always follow because this is not a perfect world but at least we can try our best by putting as much good into the world and overall the world will be a better place. During these difficult times I have seen so much good done so we can only hope the world is a better place now.

Kingsley

Fri 5 Mar

Dear Friends

Perhaps it is just me but I feel there is an air of expectancy, you all know me well enough by now to know this is normal for me. I know we still have a way to go and the present is still sad and there are difficulties ahead, yet I am excited about the prospect of what is to come. Today holds treasures we are yet to find. All through this pandemic people have had reasons to celebrate even if at a smaller gathering, there have been birthdays, anniversaries, new babies, life has gone on it is only a different life to the one we were used to before. And we know we will be able to gather again in time. The worst is over and with the coming of Easter we can look forward to a new start even if it is a gradual one. We continue to wait and reflect during this Lent, preparing our hearts and our souls for the joy that is to come.

Kingsley

Sat 6 Mar

Dear Friends

When Mike and I, and then when Jo-an and I, climbed Snowdon it took a few hours both ways. It gave us a chance to admire the views and take pictures. We climbed above the clouds and looked down at the world beneath. There is a competition to run up and down and the current record is just over an hour. That is an endurance race rather than a sightseeing amble, I wouldn't have thought they did it for pleasure but then it is a good thing we are all different. Each of us goes at our own pace in life and it is what we fill our lives with that is more important than how long we live. This pandemic, has it been an endurance for you or has it been an opportunity to slow down and look at the sights along the way? In either case it has been hard and sad and there have been joys along the way.

Because I sit here every morning and gaze out of the window for a while before I tap away at the keyboard and Jo-an and I have walked a lot I have watched the changing seasons which normally because of the pressure of the Church year I don't always notice. I have watched the phases of the moon and have discovered that each full moon has a name, the most recent being the Snow Moon. At the moment the only pressing thing is the celebration of Easter but there is no pressure to have Easter Vestry meetings. And in the world beyond the Church there is the promise of things beginning to open again at Easter but we don't yet know what. The pace of life has been so different over the last year, I hope it has taught us all to slow down and appreciate the world around us more. You will always get people who are caught up in things and will never know that the best things in life really are free. We live in a world of endless wonder so let us enjoy it, let us appreciate what we have and not strive for what we don't need.

Kingsley

Sun 7 Mar

Subject: The Third Sunday of Lent

Dear Friends

John 2. 13-22. John's gospel wasn't written as an exact historical account of his experiences with Jesus but was a well thought out proof of who Jesus was which is why it doesn't always match the other gospels. The clearing of the temple at the beginning of Jesus' ministry rather than towards the end was for a very good reason, but this is not a theological email so I won't discuss it here. However, John's mention of Jesus' mother and brothers is also deliberate to show Jesus had a normal family and was totally human as well as being God, his earthly experience is a normal one and out of this normality comes his divine mission. To suggest his mother was somehow a step away from the rest of humanity puts Jesus further away from the rest of us even more so, but John firmly grounds Jesus with us on our level. So when we go through difficult times we do not have a remote God who doesn't care, there are times when we cannot see this, times when he seems far away and we have our questions and our doubts, but he does know what it is like. Look back at my email of Sunday 5th April 2020 (page 9 in the book), this is still not a completely satisfactory answer, it is one we still wrestle with, but it is a promise.

Kingsley

Mon 8 Mar

Subject: Week 50

Dear Friends

In 1997 I was packing up my things in Llanelli preparing to come to Whitland, in those days the parish was Whitland, Cyffig and Henllan Amgoed. This was going to be my first parish as Vicar and as it has turned out my last as well, and although I haven't moved (except down into the garden) everything else has changed around me. When you have found where you are meant to be why move? After all if you are not happy where you are it doesn't mean you will be happy somewhere else because you always take yourself with you. This year the whole world has changed around us. A journey doesn't have to be from place to place because the passing of time is a journey anyway, we may not have physically moved but we are not where we were a year ago. If you go back to a place where you once lived you would not find it the same, and with the journey of time you cannot even go back except in memory. We cannot go back to the time before the pandemic, so much has changed and continues to do so. We are on a journey together, I don't just mean those I send this email to, and it is in our shared experience we have the courage to step into the future and we all contribute to whatever the future will be. As I have often said, the future is an undiscovered country, let us discover it together and marvel at the wonders it holds. Every morning I wake expecting to find something new, I wonder what today has in store.

Kingsley

Tue 9 Mar

Dear Friends

Yesterday I saw lambs in a field and I cut Jo-an's lawn, spring is definitely with us although winter can still throw some surprises at us. Spring also seems to be with us as far as the pandemic is concerned and I wonder can we hope that we won't be thrown any surprises there. We can begin to prepare for the time when the lockdown is eased and although life has gone on many things have been put on hold that we need to be picking up on. Many things perhaps we will be nervous about, we have been living under a certain amount of threat and fear and getting used to the gradual freedoms may take some getting used to. We are lucky here, when Jo-an and I have been out walking we have met people and chatted, but perhaps many people will find it strange to have a proper face to face conversation again. There are certain milestones along the way to look out for, dispensing with masks, singing, visiting each other in their homes, eating out in a restaurant, not in that order though. One day we will be able to look back at this and assess what we have done, what we have learned, and how we coped. All of life is a series of experiences that can teach us something, this is just a massive experience for all of us.

Although we can hope for the future we still live through the present, we still make the most of each day as it comes, we still look for the magic in each moment. Enjoy today with hope in your hearts.

Kingsley

Wed 10 Mar

Dear Friends

First, I was saddened to hear this morning of the passing of M H, we have been friends for a very long time and she was a valued minister in the group. Secondly, we were down in Pendine yesterday to prepare for the re-opening of the church, do they have the LMA's permission to do so?

Life is a strange thing isn't it, sadness and joy go together. I remember one strange weekend in Llanelli when I was curate. On the Saturday I was with a couple arranging a wedding in the morning, I was in the home of someone dying in the afternoon and was taken upstairs to pray just after they died, and then on the Sunday I took a Baptism. Ecclesiastes 3. 1-8. There is always light and dark, the cycle of life turns ever onward. We have a choice, we cannot always change events as they happen but we can chose how we face them. We can choose how we face the world with all its complexities, we can choose how we deal with those around us, we can choose whether we are good people or bad, we can choose whether we become bitter or understanding, we can choose to be trusting or suspicious. How are we going to face today? Are we going to let the dark drag us down or are we going to let the light shine through us. Remember, in a dark room it only takes one candle and the room is no longer dark.

Kingsley

Thu 11 Mar

Dear Friends

Either no one is a Shakespeare scholar or everyone is too polite to correct me but the Undiscovered Country quote in Hamlet is not the future but the afterlife, rather the reference to an unknown future is from Star Trek. However, I prefer to use it in the context of an unknown future because the future is more unknown than the afterlife which has been studied throughout history and we know we will be met by those we have lost when we get there, whereas the future we all go blindly into together. The second misquote is that the world is a place of Endless Wonder, I challenge you all to find out why, and there again I prefer to use it as a description of the world around us because the world really is a place of endless wonder.

The quote that God is The Maker Of All Things is Jeremiah 10.16 and 51.19, although that is not where I first heard this.

We have to be careful when we take things out of context because much harm can be done. The above examples are deliberate because the phrases I use are to convey a thought or an idea that otherwise I wouldn't be able to express properly and at least I have explained myself. After all the future is an undiscovered country that we are journeying into together, we are all explorers, the world is also a place of endless wonder and each day brings us something new and exciting. And God is The Maker Of All Things, and therefore the unknown future is also in his hands.

Kingsley

Fri 12 Mar

Dear Friends

Good news and bad news, there are some easing of restrictions in Wales however we are still only allowed to travel five miles with some flexibility in rural areas and although we are in a rural area the Cathedral would be stretching it a little so the Pilgrim Service planned for 10th of April will have to be postponed, please let everyone know.

As we come over the brow of the hill we realise that our destination is a little further away than we thought, but it is still there in the distance. This time is a balancing act for our leaders and there will be some people who say the easing is too fast and others who say it is too slow. It is what it is and we must be sensible. This probably means that these emails will continue longer than I was beginning to think, though I still intend to submit them to the publisher just after Easter and hope there will not be a third book.

God's plans are always long term plans, his promise of saving the world took thousands of years, when Jesus was eventually born he still had to grow up and it is thought he was about 30 when he began his ministry. The Israelites were forty years in the wilderness before entering the Promised Land. We tend to expect instant replies, when we text someone we can get an answer in seconds, when I email the Archdeacon with a Risk Assessment I usually get it back the next day, when we pray to God we have no idea if and when we will get a reply. There is a saying 'God isn't sleeping', he is working through his plans and perhaps we will only recognise his hand in things afterwards. Keep the faith, hold on to hope, live in joy.

Kingsley

Sat 13 Mar

Dear Friends

In the early church lent was a period of excitement and hope, new converts to Christianity were being taught all they needed to know about their new faith and the rest of the church prayed for them ready to welcome them into the fellowship at Easter. Traditionally there are no flowers in Church during lent and I have been unable to find a good reason for this, it is spring after all and the world outside the church is ablaze with flowers, and this is God's world and God's doing, why does the church somehow deem it wrong to display flowers? Jesus often grumbled at the Jewish authorities because of their tradition rather than caring for people. I wonder if this is another Roman tradition and perhaps the Celtic Church being much closer to nature and seeing spirituality in the world that God created didn't ban flowers, here I am speculating. The wilderness where Jesus spent forty days was not a desert and there would have been flowers blooming there. The world is not an evil place that we should cut ourselves off from, evil does not come from outside but from within our own hearts and thoughts if we let it, there is evil out there but we have been given the power to resist it. Bad things happen in the world but how much of this is because of the people in it. If we look for fault we can always feel hard done by, if we seek to do good, if there is good in our hearts, then we add to the good in the world. Make the world a better place today.

Kingsley

P.S.

Holy Week and Easter

Mon 29 Mar 2.30 pm Short meditation at St Brynach's Llanboidy

Tue 30 Mar 2.30 pm Short meditation at St David's Clunderwen

Maundy Thursday 1 Apr 2.30 pm Eucharist at Cyffig

Good Friday 2 Apr 11.00 am Hour meditation at St Tysilio's Llandysilio

Easter Sunday 4 Apr 10.30 am Eucharist at St Brybach's Llanboidy with Jeni and 11.00 am Eucharist at St Mary's Whitland with me

Sun 14 Mar

Subject: The Fourth Sunday of Lent/Mothering Sunday

Dear Friends

Luke 2. 33-35. Joseph and Mary take the baby Jesus to the temple, here Simeon blesses him and says the piece that is known as the Nunc Dimitis. The short reading for today comes immediately after, Jesus' parents marvel at what is said, Simeon blesses them, pronounces a further prophecy and warns Mary "And a sword will pierce your own soul too." For Mary would be a witness to his crucifixion. Sometimes God expects an awful lot of people, Mary was not a super being, she was not somehow distanced from all other mothers by some divine grace, she was a simple Jewish woman and this was going to hurt her deeply. Did she really need to know this at the beginning? It would be a dark cloud that would haunt her all her life. No wonder she asked him to come away from the crowds later in his ministry.

We know that Jesus was fully human and felt all the feelings we feel, the joys and the sorrows. We know he had a human heart and should understand just how fragile it can be. But he knew he had a destiny, a purpose to fulfil, does he fully understand that we do not know even when God does have a destiny for us. We struggle through life trying to make sense of it, at times desperately hanging on to our small faith. There are times in Jesus' life he appears to take his mother for granted and yet practically his last thought on the cross was of her, that she should be looked after. God does care, if only he made it more obvious at times because we have so many questions.

Kingsley

Mon 15 Mar

Subject: Week 51

Dear Friends

When I was in Theological College we took it in turns to take Morning or Evening Prayer, it was part of the training and we were still learning. However no one told us if we did it right, we only knew because no one told us what mistakes we had made, occasionally I would make a mistake just to get some feedback. Very often people are very quick to find fault or criticise so it is always a nice surprise to be complimented for something. At this point in the pandemic peoples nerves are getting a little frayed and perhaps a little quick to snap because we can see the light on the horizon and are somewhat frustrated that we still have to wait for the dawn. Because these are unusual times our lives don't have the structure we are used to and haven't for such a long time now. I enjoy this time in the morning, quietly gazing out of the window and tapping away at the computer, it gives my day some structure. When things begin to slowly return to some semblance of normal we will have to learn to do the simple things we took for granted again, having had the space to assess what is important and what is not.

Easter is a time of renewal and rebirth, as Easter approaches let us get ourselves ready for it even if it is only tentative at first. Easter will not be the end of the lockdown just the beginning of greater freedom, let us appreciate each new freedom in turn. Today, just take a moment to find peace within yourself.

Kingsley

Tue 16 Mar

Dear Friends

Just to repeat what I said in an earlier email, the Pilgrim Service in the Cathedral has been postponed. This is sad because I had hoped to have this near enough to the anniversary of my daily emails, before this they were not daily just keeping in touch. I have appreciated your willingness to read my daily rambling thoughts and I have enjoyed the replies I get, this has been a lifeline in the storm. When I mention the book to people it is hard to explain what it is about, it is not thoughts for the day although I hope it has been encouraging, there is no structure or plan but it is a window into how my mind works and a glimpse of things I am interested in and I am humbled to find that people read them every day. For future historians these will be a glimpse of what it was like to live through this time as first book is (and the second will be) deposited in the major libraries of the UK, otherwise future generations will not know what it has been like for us who are living through it. Life has been strange, we have lost so much in many ways, but life has gone on. We have all found ways to carry on, to cope with the sadness, and even to find joy. We have all learned many lessons during this time and I hope discovered strengths in ourselves we didn't know we had. Our faith has been tested and we are still no nearer answers than we were at the beginning, but we continue with hope. We look to a bright future and continue to live for today, looking for the wonders and magic each day has to offer. Go boldly into today with a song in your heart.

Kingsley

Wed 17 Mar

Dear Friends

Happy St. Patrick's Day. An interesting and little known fact is that although he is venerated as a Saint in the Catholic Church he was never formally canonised because he lived before the current laws in this matter, here we go again, official church laws. Who really cares? He was a missionary, he saw miracles, he changed people's lives, even if we can't pin him down to an exact date his work in Ireland has lasted and surely that is what really matters. Life is not tidy, it doesn't fit into neat boxes, good does not work to a timetable or official rules. If we waited for a committee or set up a foundation to do good works, to care for people, nothing would get done. Some people like to talk about things without actually getting round to it. Isn't it good that there are so many people who do not wait, who do not talk, but act, people who see a need and simply do something. So many people in this world have done so much good without having to be officially recognised by the Catholic Church, their recognition is by God.

Today let us just get on with life, do the good things and help wherever we can, and overall the world will be a better place.

Kingsley

Thu 18 Mar

Dear Friends

The 1945 film of Blythe Spirit begins "When we are young we read and believe the most fantastic things. When we grow older and wiser we learn, perhaps with a little regret, that these things can never be." I am afraid I never grew older and certainly not wiser. Children have a way understanding things with simplicity and wonder that many adults lose, and why? Sometimes perhaps because life can be hard, more often because they would appear to be foolish, and perhaps what we call our rational mind dismisses them. And what is faith if not a belief in fantastic things? How often do we almost catch sight of something and our rational mind quickly steps in and says it cannot be, how often do we hear faint music with no source and shut our ears to it. How often do our hearts burn within us like the people on the road to Emmaus and we dismiss it. If we lose wonder our lives lack colour.

At the moment, as the pandemic drags on, now we need wonder and magic more than ever. We need to be able to lift our spirits out of the stress and the fear and soar as only our spirits can. There are no restrictions on dreams and hopes, our souls do not need to socially distance, and our inner selves need no masks.

Kingsley

Fri 19 Mar

Dear Friends

There are a finite number of notes yet the amount of music seems endless, there are only 26 letters in the alphabet yet the stories and the thoughts that are expressed will never stop, the visible spectrum is quite short yet the art that uses is it will go on. There is no end to imagination and inspiration. Our world is a place of endless wonder and there are always new things to see, new experiences, new people to meet, new things to find. For many people this last year has been hard because they couldn't go out and have had to rely on others bringing news and supplies, technology being their window on the world, but it is amazing what you can see through a window. The changing of the seasons, the varied weather, the comings and goings of people.

When we have greater freedom we must all live life to the full again, appreciate all that we have and no longer take anything for granted. And even today holds unexpected surprises let us look forward to what they are.

Kingsley

Sat 20 Mar

Dear Friends

Today is the Spring Equinox, when days and nights are the same length, and the alignment of St Mary's Churchyard is with the rising sun. The Neolithic people aligned it that way because they understood the cycle of life and that death was but a gateway into the Otherworld, they also understood the need to mark significant positions of the sun because they were farmers and farming has to keep track of the changing seasons. The whole of life revolved around an understanding of the natural world and enclosures (which we refer to as henges) such as the one where St Mary's is were important for so many reasons. It was a calendar to mark the seasons, it was a centre for worship, it was a place to celebrate the coming together of two people, the birth of a child and the passing of a loved one, and as a church it still serves the same purpose. Because God The Maker Of All Things designed the world as it is from the beginning and we are a part of that creation and live in it, what is truly amazing is that he chose to live in it and become wholly part of it too. Appreciate the natural world around us, see it as a place of endless wonder, live in it and rejoice with each new day.

Kingsley

Sun 21 Mar

Subject: Passion Sunday

Dear Friends

John 12. 20-33. Jesus is approaching the time of his crucifixion and he warns his disciples what to expect and faces them with a choice. He has come to the point in his ministry when he must die so that he is no longer just one voice, he must fulfil what he came for to save everyone. And the choice for us is to either seek to look after ourselves only and in the end lose everything or be willing to give ourselves to help others and gain everything. I often wonder what happened to the Greeks who wished to see him at the beginning of this passage, John doesn't say, Jesus never turned anyone away so I can only assume they did get to see him. In any case because of his death and resurrection we all have access to him, we do not have a remote God who looks down on humanity and expects us to do as we are told but a God who shares our humanity and lived by example, the choice then is up to us. Do we selfishly only think of ourselves or do we have compassion on others and want to help. Thankfully as we have seen very much in evidence throughout this pandemic there are so many people who have been willing to put the interests of others before themselves, the NHS, the key workers, the individuals who have done so much for the isolated, there is a goodness in humanity that far outweighs the bad.

Kingsley

Mon 22 Mar

Subject: Week 52

Dear Friends

Two things we need at the moment, a sense of perspective and a sense of humour. This is a worldwide pandemic so many people have died and everyone is hurting, no one is unaffected, we have to address that and cannot just brush it off. This has been and still is a massive event in all our lives and we need to be there for each other rather than hide ourselves away, family, friends, community and those we are responsible to are how we get through this together. Being wrapped up in ourselves doesn't help anyone, especially not ourselves, to help ourselves we need to help others.

And a sense of humour. Laughter is a great gift. I have never really taken myself too seriously which is just as well because I can be quite intense at times. To be able to see the funny side of things is not to diminish the importance of something but it does break the tension and in a strange way does affect our sense of perspective. To be able to laugh and smile through adversity keeps us sane.

And above all, keep your eyes open to the wonders of the world around you, live with hope and joy.

Kingsley

Tue 23 Mar

Subject: One Year

Dear Friends

A year since the first lockdown in the UK, did any of us expect to be where we are now? A year since we lost our old normal and we have lived through so many changes of the rules it has been hard to keep up. And now we have come to realise that we won't get our old normal back for a long time. We knew things would change and now it has sunk in just how much has changed. The one thing that hit me the most was the edict that not only were the churches to close but that I was not even allowed to enter a church! I had planned to go down to St Mary's, ring the bell, and pray every day which I had been doing up until this point, and then to be denied that and where was the harm? 'Stay Home, Protect the NHS, Save lives.' and most of us did. But then the sun was shining and it was as if the whole of nature rested.

Each of us has dealt with this in our own way and some better than others. Today we pause and reflect, we pray for all who have died, we give thanks to those who have gone above and beyond, we have compassion for all who have suffered in mind, body and spirit. We draw a breath and march on into the future with hope.

Kingsley

Wed 24 Mar

Dear Friends

I have two dragons, they are in jars with a piece of hessian tied over the top. They are quiet and still at the moment but the label warns that they should be kept out of direct sunlight and I should not remove the cover. Such is the way with dragons that if I were to let them out they would immediately become full sized and would rampage over the countryside. So I am very careful to leave them alone in a bright airy place. The trouble with people is that they tend to let dragons out of jars, Adam did and humanity has borne the brunt, the present virus is an example of letting the dragon out of the jar. Where is the red dragon when we need him? The red dragon is the people who have worked tirelessly to cope with the pandemic and those who have developed a vaccine. The dragon will become less fierce with time and we will learn to live with it.

Easter is when Jesus defeated the ancient dragon, and although he still roams about he has no teeth and we live with hope and the knowledge that even death is not the end.

Kingsley

Thu 25 Mar

Dear Friends

A year ago today I sent the first email, I didn't have many addresses to send it to, just over twenty. It was just to tell everyone I was here if needed and mostly it was a quote from a book I was reading. It wasn't going to be a daily email but it was a seed. It was the first step along a journey, a journey that is still going a year later. We have been through joy and sorrow together, hard stretches and easy patches, celebration and loss. Our hopes have been raised and dashed and raised again.

Last year we could not celebrate Easter, this year we can but tentatively, people are still cautious. There is no pressure on people to do what they are afraid to do, we are only coming out of this latest lockdown cautiously, with one eye on a possible third wave. But we must not be too afraid to live, even in the darkest hours there are stars in the sky and the sun is only hiding round the other side of the world - those of you in Australia can see him when we can't. Those of us with hope owe it to those who don't to give comfort and assurance. Together we are strong.

Kingsley

Fri 26 Mar

Dear Friends

Do you have dreams? Over time have you let go or forgotten dreams you once had? Were your dreams reasonable in the first place? This year particularly has taken its toll on dreams we may have had, perhaps our dreams are simpler now. To be able to go on holiday, to go out for a meal, to meet up with family and friends, to cwtch, to sing. Yet we shouldn't ever give up on our dreams even the seemingly unreasonable ones, they may still happen. This is a strange world and the twists and turns of life can take us into unexpected places, if we stop looking we will never find, if we stop expecting we will never be surprised. We may never be rich and famous for they are vastly overrated and do not bring happiness or contentment. Yet dreams do take shape. Never stop looking at the world as a child does, never stop seeing wonder in everything, never stop dreaming.

Kingsley

Sat 27 Mar

Dear Friends

I am looking forward to going back into all of my five churches next week for Holy Week meditations, some of them I only briefly went in to last summer to prepare for the risk assessment, this is going to be an emotional journey for me. Many things we are all going to find emotional as slowly we are given more freedom in the next months. Today in Wales we can travel as far as we like, libraries are open, outdoor places of historical interest and gardens are open, sport for under 18's. I will probably do what I did yesterday, I have no plans to go anywhere, but I am sure many people will enjoy the greater freedom. There will also be many people still too afraid or cautious to venture out much, we must be gentle with ourselves and only do what we are comfortable with, and the virus is still with us.

Our journey continues and I have no plans to stop writing. Today through my window the sun is shining and the sky is blue, the grass is growing and I must cut it soon, the rooks are building their nests very high in the trees and I hope this is a good sign for the summer. I haven't seen so many people walking past since the schools have gone back, but next week is the Easter break so I expect the Roman Road will be busy, except people can go further afield now. This truly is spring, tonight the hour changes, our lives begin to open up again and we can move forward with joy.

Kingsley

Part 12
Easter

Sun 28 Mar

Subject: Palm Sunday

Dear Friends

Mark 11. 1-11. Jesus enters Jerusalem, people spread cloaks on the road or branches they had cut in the fields, they shouted "Hosanna!" and acknowledged him as the son of David. This was a glorious moment and I often wonder what Jesus thought at this moment, because in a few days they would shout "Crucify him.", yet this was his whole purpose in coming to Jerusalem, the whole point of being born into the world. Holy Week can be very intense if you take the trouble to live through it examining what Jesus was doing day by day. I will never forget Holy Week when I was in Theological College, the University was on break so we concentrated on the events of the week, something I haven't been able to recapture in the parish. Last year we were in complete lockdown and my only opportunity was my own reflections and my emails which had suddenly become daily, this year I can celebrate Holy Week by going into the five churches of my group. Whatever our own struggles at this time for Jesus and his disciples this was the pivotal point of all history. Let this be a pivotal point in our history too, we live through difficult days in order to come through to rejoice again.

"Blessed is he who comes in the name of the Lord!"

Kingsley

Mon 29 Mar

Subject: Monday in Holy Week

Dear Friends

In Matthews Gospel early the next day Jesus was hungry and passing a fig tree found nothing but leaves and cursed the tree so it died. This does seem rather unlike him, yet if everything he did was for a purpose and an opportunity to give a message then it is what he says after that important. He talks about the faith to move mountains and to receive whatever you ask in prayer. And this has always been a problem for us because I am sure that everyone has prayed ardently for something in their lives and believed strongly, and yet have known disappointment. Is our faith not strong enough? Do we not understand the will of God? This will remain for me one of those questions I do not really have an answer for. And then again, sometimes our prayers are answered in the most unexpected ways. We must hold on to faith, but it also requires an awful lot of trust on our behalf that God will answer in his way even when we can't see it ourselves.

Kingsley

Tue 30 Mar

Subject: Tuesday in Holy Week

Dear Friends

Many of the parables Jesus used at this time were directed at the Jewish authorities knowing full well they were rejecting him and the miracles he performed made no difference, his message was therefore for the ordinary people who would listen. There will always be those who have made up their minds already, usually those full of their own importance, and nothing you can say or do will change that. To hear the message we must be humble and open, ready to listen and receive the good news. The authorities in Jesus time had too much to lose, but where are they now? You cannot hold on to power and authority and wealth after you die. Not even the Pharaohs could take their wealth with them despite the lengths they went to with their tombs, their wealth was taken either by robbers or archaeologists. True treasure is not measured in wealth or status but honesty of heart, in the humility to accept the free gift that Jesus has won for us. Holy Week is all about the choice we face, to care only for ourselves or care for others, to hold on to what we have or to give freely that we may receive a greater reward.

Kingsley

Wed 31 Mar

Subject: Wednesday in Holy Week

Dear Friends

While walking round Jerusalem Jesus' disciples draw his attention to the buildings, particularly the temple, perhaps some of them hadn't been there before. Jesus is not impressed and says that it will be destroyed. This leads his disciples to ask about the end of the age, he tells them about the difficult times that will come such as wars and rumours of wars, he tells them about deceptions such as people claiming to be him, he warns them about suffering and persecution, and about the end when he will return in glory and with the angels. Throughout history people have analysed this to predict the end of the world and I expect the present pandemic has featured in that, but the world has not ended yet despite the number of times is was supposed to have. Jesus doesn't give a timescale, he warns that we will not know, people will be going about their daily lives as normal, therefore we should all be prepared at all times. We must also remember this is only a very small part of what Jesus said, the vast majority of his teaching is about living in the present. We should be concerned with life now not what may or may not happen. It is what we do from day to day, our caring for one another, our witness of our faith, our enjoying the world that God has given us and our appreciation of all our blessings that is what matters.

Kingsley

Thu 1 Apr

Subject: Maundy Thursday

Dear Friends

Jesus shares his last supper with his disciples, although it is not the last time he eats with them as he does so after his resurrection. It is when he instigates the meal we commemorate as Communion or Eucharist and in this act we are invited to share his last supper with him. It is when he links the breaking of bread and drinking of wine with his sacrifice of torn body and spilled blood. It is when he reminds his disciples that he is as at one time God and servant by washing their feet. It is when he speaks of betrayal and sends Judas out into the dark. And after supper he prays in anguish in the garden and accepts the will of his Father. The spiritual battle he fought within himself was won this evening. So much happened this evening that is of such great importance to us as Christians and yet I have never had many at a Maundy Thursday service. Can we not wait with him one hour?

Kingsley

Fri 2 Apr

Subject: Good Friday

Dear Friends

I will be in St Tysilio's for the Hour Meditation this morning and don't know what I will find to say for a whole hour, although some of it will be taken up with recorded hymns (we still can't sing). Today is the important day for Christianity, it is the day Jesus took away sin and died in our place, it is sad that so many people want to hang on to sin and will not let him take it. The power of death has been destroyed but it still affects us all because it separates us from our loved ones. Satan has been defeated but he still prowls around. The victory Jesus gained is something we have to grasp, we have to turn from the darkness and face the light, we have to accept as a free gift the life he offers. The choice is ours, sin or goodness, dark or light, death or life, he has opened up the way but it is us who must walk in it.

Kingsley

Sat 3 Apr

Subject: Easter Eve

Dear Friends

The Saturday between Good Friday and Easter Sunday is always a strange day for us as we go through the stages of Holy Week and Easter, it is a day for reflection. For the disciples it was devastating and frightening. Their teacher who they had followed and had begun to realise he was the promised Messiah had been executed and was buried, their purpose and their hopes dashed, and there was the constant fear that the authorities wouldn't stop there and they faced the threat of arrest and death.

This week has been a journey for me, I have been round all my five churches now, some I haven't taken a service in for over a year, and met up with people I haven't seen for a year either. We have reflected and meditated and we have chatted, it has been a good week and I am grateful to those who attended. Today also marks the anniversary of my second email which still wasn't a daily one, then I was asking if anyone knew the emails of people who I could contact and little did I suspect just how far reaching these ramblings would become.

So, today we sit back and reflect, preparing our hearts and minds for Easter, and see what unexpected things today brings.

Kingsley

Sun 4 Apr

Subject: Easter Day

Dear Friends

Christ is risen Alleluia!

Today is the fulfilment of God's eternal plan, the day all sin is forgiven through Jesus' sacrifice, the chasm between us and God has been crossed and the way to eternal life is open. We simply have to admit our sin, ask for and receive forgiveness. It is the day of new life and new hope.

In nature around us there are blossoms on bushes and trees, new leaves are beginning to open with the fresh green of spring.

For us today the lockdown is slowly easing but we still have a long way to go. Let us face today with joy because it is a new day and it will bring blessing.

Happy Easter

Kingsley

Mon 5 Apr

Subject: The end?

Dear Friends

I have written a circular email every day for a year now, I have been back to all my five churches through Holy Week and I have celebrated Easter in St Mary's, now would be a good time to stop. We have been through so much together, loss, sadness, dark days and long hauls. There has also been much to celebrate and be thankful for, and there has been joy along the way. I am grateful to you for your support through it all and still can't get over that my ramblings have spread so far, thank-you for being willing to share my thoughts.

Today is a day for hope, the vaccine is rolling out, the number of infections and deaths have dropped considerably, and there are gradual easing of restrictions. The world has changed, our ways of doing many things are different now, we have all learned new things. We have reflected and reassessed, we have faced ourselves. And now we must look to the future, having come through hard times we have the courage to face whatever is ahead. Be brave, rejoice in the small things, live confidently.

So, is this goodbye? No.

Kingsley